Engaging Patients as Safety Partners

Engaging Patients as Safety Partners

A Guide for Reducing Errors and Improving Satisfaction

Patrice L. Spath

Editor

Health Forum, Inc.
An American Hospital Association Company
CHICAGO

AHA
press

Portions of this book were published in earlier form in *Partnering with Patients to Reduce Medical Errors,* edited by Patrice L. Spath (Chicago: Health Forum, Inc., 2004).

𝖠𝖧𝖠 is a service mark of the American Hospital Association used under license by AHA Press.

Printed in the United States of America—06/08

Cover design by Cheri Kusek

ISBN: 978-1-55648-353-0   Item Number: 181203

Library of Congress Cataloging-in-Publication Data

Engaging patients as safety partners : a guide for reducing errors and improving satisfaction / Patrice L. Spath, editor.
    p. ; cm.
Includes bibliographical references and index.
ISBN 978-1-55648-353-0 (alk. paper)
    1. Medical errors—Prevention. 2. Patient satisfaction. 3. Patient participation. 4. Medicine—Safety measures. I. Spath, Patrice.
    [DNLM: 1. Hospitals. 2. Medical Errors—prevention & control. 3. Models, Organizational. 4. Patient Participation. 5. Safety Management—methods. WX 153 E565 2008]
    R729.8.E54 2008
    362.1068—dc22
                2008002216

*This book is lovingly dedicated
to my son, Gordon Spath,
and my daughter, Karen Fine.*

Contents

List of Figures and Table

About the Editor

Patrice L. Spath, BA, RHIT, is a health information management professional with broad experience in health care quality and resource management. During the past 25 years, she has presented more than 300 educational programs on performance improvement, case management, and patient safety improvement topics. She has also authored numerous books and journal articles on these subjects.

Ms. Spath has extensive knowledge of patient safety improvement techniques. She has authored and edited several books on this topic, including *Error Reduction in Health Care: A Systems Approach to Improving Patient Safety* (Jossey-Bass/AHA Press, 2000), *Partnering with Patients to Reduce Medical Errors* (AHA Press, 2004), and *101 Tools for Improving Health Care Performance* (Brown-Spath & Associates, 2005). She can be reached at www.brownspath.com.

Ms. Spath serves on the advisory board for *WebM&M*, an online, case-based journal and forum on patient safety and health care quality sponsored by the Agency for Healthcare Research and Quality (http://webmm.ahrq.gov).

About the Contributors

Geraldine (Geri) Amori, PhD, ARM, CPHRM, DFASHRM, is senior director of education and professional development for the Risk Management and Patient Safety Institute, Lansing, Michigan (www.rmpsi.com). She is a board member of Consumers Advancing Patient Safety, an adviser to the Partnership for Patient Safety, and a lifetime member of the American Society for Healthcare Risk Management.

Kay Beauregard, RN, MSA, is administrative director of Royal Oak Beaumont Hospital, Royal Oak, Michigan. The Beaumont Hospitals in Royal Oak and Troy were finalists for the 2003 American Hospital Quest for Quality Prize.

Cindy Brach, MPP, is a senior health policy researcher at the Agency for Healthcare Research and Quality (AHRQ), where she spearheads AHRQ's health literacy activities, coordinating AHRQ's work in developing measures and improving the evidence base, and integrating health literacy activities throughout AHRQ's portfolios.

Maggie M. Finkelstein, Esquire, is an attorney in private practice affiliated with the law practice of Stevens & Lee, Lancaster, Pennsylvania. Her practice is concentrated in health law, with a focus on loss control and event management for physicians and health care organizations. She is a member of the American Health Lawyers Association and regularly publishes on loss control and risk management topics.

Cezanne Garcia, MPH, CHES, is associate director of patient- and family-centered care and education at the University of

Washington Medical Center, Seattle, where she directs a broad range of patient- and family-centered care improvement and patient education programs that actively engage patients, families, and staff in collaborative partnerships.

Joel Mattison, MD, FACS, a board-certified plastic and reconstructive surgeon, is the former medical director of clinical resource management at St. Joseph's Hospital in Tampa, Florida. During his tenure, Dr. Mattison established and edited *Off the Record,* a monthly newsletter intended to improve communication among physicians at the hospital.

Michelle H. Pelling, MBA, RN, is a health care management consultant and president of the ProPell Group, Newberg, Oregon (www.propellgroup.com). She is the author of *Hospital Manager's Guide to Joint Commission Standards* and co-author of *Outcomes Management: Using Data to Improve Decision Making.*

Thomas C. Royer, MD, is president and chief executive officer of CHRISTUS Health, a Catholic health care system consisting of forty hospitals and long-term care facilities in Texas, Arkansas, Louisiana, Oklahoma, Utah, and Mexico. The system is headquartered in Irving, Texas.

James W. Saxton, Esquire, is an attorney in private practice affiliated with the law practice of Stevens & Lee, Lancaster, Pennsylvania. He is co-chair of the firm's Health Care Department and chair of the firm's Health Care Litigation Group. He is also the immediate past chair of the American Health Lawyers Association's Healthcare Liability and Litigation Group. He speaks nationally on health care and risk management issues.

Paula S. Swain, RN, MSN, CPHQ, FNAHQ, is director of clinical and regulatory review at Presbyterian Hospital in Charlotte, North Carolina. She is also president of Swain and Associates, a firm specializing in health care quality improvement and compliance consulting and training (www.snaconsulting.com).

Robert M. Wachter, MD, is professor and associate chairman, department of medicine; chief of the division of hospital medicine; and chair of the Patient Safety Committee, University of California, San Francisco. Dr. Wachter is the editor of the Agency for Healthcare Research and Quality's online journals *WebM&M* and *Patient Safety Network*. He is the lead author of *Internal Bleeding: The Truth behind America's Terrifying Epidemic of Medical Mistakes* (Rugged Land, 2004) and the author of *Understanding Patient Safety* (McGraw-Hill, 2008).

Steven Winokur, MD, is medical director, quality improvement, and chief patient safety officer at Royal Oak Beaumont Hospital, Royal Oak, Michigan. The Beaumont Hospitals in Royal Oak and Troy were finalists for the 2003 American Hospital Quest for Quality Prize.

Theresa M. Zimmerman, RN, BSN, JD, ARM, CPHRM, is the divisional patient safety officer for Catholic Healthcare Partners, headquartered in Cincinnati, Ohio. She is past president of the Ohio Society of Healthcare Risk Management and currently serves on the board of directors for the American Society for Healthcare Risk Management.

Foreword

Robert M. Wachter, MD

Before my book, *Internal Bleeding,* came out in 2004, the publisher hired a media coach to prepare me for what we hoped would be many radio and television appearances promoting the book.[1] The media game is easy, my coach assured me, once you appreciate a few tricks of the trade. Answer the question *you* want to answer, not necessarily the one that was asked. Use vivid, dramatic examples. And most of all: Keep it Short and Simple, Stupid.

The training was useful, and during the scores of interviews I have done in the past several years on patient safety topics, I have generally stuck to the script: "Did you realize, Kathy, that in the thirty minutes you've been on the air today, five Americans died of medical mistakes?" That sort of thing.

But there was one question that always seemed to derail my Talking Point Express, and it was the one question that I could count on being asked in virtually every interview, long or short, TV or radio, sophisticated interviewer or one not so sophisticated: "Tell me, Doc," it always began, "what can patients do to protect themselves?"

Why would this question, whose answer seems so obvious, throw me wildly off message? Surely, the virtues of an informed patient or family, able to participate in their own medical decisions, are unassailable. Moreover, from a patient safety perspective, an extra set of eyes primed to notice and empowered to point out hazards ("Nurse, the medicine you just gave me has another person's name on it." "Doctor, I didn't see you wash your hands when you entered the room.") will surely prevent medical errors periodically. Asking for proof of the virtues of these commonsensical interventions might be like seeking proof of the value of parachutes, as was described in a *British Medical Journal* satirical shiv aimed at the heart of evidence-based medicine ideologues.[2]

Parachutes notwithstanding, consider these challenges to the premise that patients can and should be central players in efforts to prevent medical mistakes:

1. Some safety and human factors engineers believe that having a patient or family member try to insert himself or herself in a complex medical process is as likely to cause confusion as to ensure safety.[3] In the early days of "sign your site," before the process was standardized by the Joint Commission, many patients tried to do their part by marking their own limbs prior to reporting for surgery. There was one problem: some patients marked the limb to be operated on, and others marked the limb to be avoided. As you might imagine, this kind of variability introduces new possibilities for errors.

2. Even if the well-informed and alert patient or loved one *can* help prevent errors, too many patients lack the resources to act as advocates for their own safety. Particularly in the hospital, many patients are confused, anxious, or sedated or have language differences, health literacy challenges, or no involved family members. This variability means that relying on a strategy of patient engagement will always be an inconsistent proposition—perhaps working when the conditions are right but falling flat too frequently to be a consistent safety bulwark.

3. Some patients and families, intent on doing what they can to prevent errors, will cross the very thin line that separates being empowered and appropriately skeptical from being angry and confrontational. The latter attitude can lead providers to adopt a defensive stance or even generate outright avoidance. I have seen nurses and doctors bypass a patient's hospital room rather than subject themselves to a mini-deposition by entering. Such a scenario does not enhance patient safety.

4. With the emphasis on patient engagement and empowerment has come some recent evidence that patients and families often feel guilty about errors, thinking that they should have done something to prevent them.[4] This is analogous to the old saw that cancer patients can prevent recurrences by thinking positively, a nice concept unless the cancer recurs, after which some suffering patients blame themselves for not thinking positively enough.

Even with these caveats, certain patient engagement strategies *do* have parachute-like face validity. Much of the progress in patient safety in the past decade has come from the involvement of patients and their proxies at a policy level. This advocacy is most vividly illustrated by those patients and families who have channeled their grief over a devastating medical error into working with the system to improve safety—a heartrending act of charity and a positive force for change. And patient engagement at an organizational level (such as having patients on key safety committees) seems likely to help keep systems focused and honest. Finally, the ethical imperative to inform patients about their care and allow them to fully participate in decisions about it is self-evident.

As I have reflected on my own ambivalence on the patient engagement issue (and why my answers to questions about it fit better on a subway trip than an elevator ride), I have found that it partly flows from the pragmatic concerns I have outlined above. But I have come to realize that it also stems from a fundamental question embedded in the premise itself: Why *should* it fall to patients and family members to ensure their own safety? When I step onto an airplane, I know that there isn't anything I can do to prevent the majority of errors that might result in my demise. When I fly, though, my feelings of impotence are trumped by my knowledge that the appropriate steps have been taken to ensure my safety. Judging by commercial aviation's remarkable safety record, this confidence is reasonably well founded. And so I relax.

Patients encountering the health care system enjoy no such trust, which makes relaxation and passivity seem like maladaptive responses, in Darwinian terms. Given this lack of trust, I cannot argue with their desire to do what they can to improve their odds of coming out alive. I have felt it myself, both as a patient and as a family member. I am just not sure how well the resulting tactics work or how to apply them most effectively. Clearly, there is a need for high-quality information on this topic.

The role of writings on patient engagement, then, is a keen topic of interest. Much of this literature tends toward the moralistic and politically correct, seeming to ask, Who would dare to question this strategy? To my mind, explorations of this complex topic need to be rigorous; thoughtful in their depiction of best practices; guided when possible by evidence; and cognizant of the subtleties, nuances, and risks. *Engaging Patients as Safety Partners,* edited by one of the world's leading patient safety authorities, navigates these challenging waters with great skill and purpose. That is why this book will be such a useful resource for patients, families, advocates, providers, and others working to prevent harm from medical errors.

In the final analysis, we are in a race—on the one hand to develop strategies and resources that truly do allow patients to help ensure their own safety and on the other hand to create a healthcare system in which patient engagement to prevent medical mistakes becomes unnecessary, a vestige of a previously flawed system. It makes no difference to me which side wins this race, as long as one of them does.

References

1. R. M. Wachter and K. G. Shojania, *Internal Bleeding: The Truth behind America's Terrifying Epidemic of Medical Mistakes* (New York: Rugged Land, 2004).
2. G. C. S. Smith and J. P. Pell, "Parachute Use to Prevent Death and Major Trauma Related to Gravitational Challenge: Systematic Review of Randomised Controlled Trials," *British Medical Journal* 327 (2003): 1459–61.
3. M. Lyons, "Should Patients Have a Role in Patient Safety? A Safety Engineering View," *Quality and Safety in Health Care* 16 (2007): 140–42.
4. T. Delbanco and S. K. Bell, "Guilty, Afraid, and Alone—Struggling with Medical Error," *New England Journal of Medicine* 357 (2007): 1682–23.

Preface

The need to avoid errors in the provision of health services is a major concern across all sites of health care delivery. Reports from the Institute of Medicine (IOM) in 1999 and 2001 emphasized the extent of harm that results from mistakes and the gap that still exists in the quality of care that people receive compared with the quality of care the system is capable of providing. The 1999 IOM report, *To Err Is Human: Building a Safer Health System,* put patient safety squarely in the forefront of the nation's health care agenda.

The second IOM report, *Crossing the Quality Chasm: A New Health System for the 21st Century* (2001), called for a transformation of the health care system to one that is patient centered, safe, effective, and equitable. Patient-centeredness has been described in a variety of ways. Essential to each definition is the realization that practitioners and organizations must respond to patient-identified needs and concerns and create higher levels of patient satisfaction with the care experience.

In 2003, when I first began to identify authors for *Partnering with Patients to Reduce Medical Errors* (AHA Press, 2004) the health care industry was just starting to embrace the patient as a partner in the safety movement. The Joint Commission, the American Hospital Association, and other national groups had developed consumer "Speak Up" campaigns to encourage caregivers and patients to collaborate for safety; however, many providers were not enthusiastically embracing these efforts. Only a few organizations on the cutting edge of safety improvement were actively partnering with patients and their family members to reduce errors.

In 2003, research studies were just getting under way to determine the value of consumer involvement in patient safety. Many questions remained unanswered. Can consumers be effective safety partners? Can they recognize risky health care situations, and will they speak up to help prevent an adverse event? What is the best way to engage patients and family members as safety partners? Will collaborating with patients and family members actually improve safety?

Sometime between 2003 and today, the proverbial "tipping point" was reached. The notion that patients and family members can have a positive impact on safety began to catch on among providers. We are now seeing a true culture shift—both within organizations and among individual caregivers. This change is attributable only in part to accreditation and regulatory requirements. Probably the greatest influencing factor has been the voice of the consumer.

When health care organizations actively share safety information with consumers, patient satisfaction scores often go up. When providers disclose medical errors to patients and family members, litigation may be avoided. When a patient or family member speaks up and a wrong-site surgery or medication error is averted, the value of safety partnerships is confirmed. Since 2003, we've learned that active collaboration with patients and families is a vital element in an organization's patient safety improvement effort.

How this collaboration occurs still varies among organizations. Some are at the "wary" stage—safety information is shared with patients, but there is little active discussion of safety issues by frontline staff during the provision of care. Many are at the "informed" stage—patients and families receive information, and during the delivery of care staff members reinforce the importance of the safety partnership through their words and actions. A few organizations are at the "forward thinking" stage. These organizations not only are sharing information and actively partnering with patients but they've also formed patient advisory groups to solicit safety improvement suggestions.

Some organizations have added former patients or community members to their patient safety committee. Some are inviting patients or family members to participate in sentinel event investigations and proactive safety improvement projects. A lot has changed since *Partnering with Patients to Reduce Medical Errors* was published, and hence I saw the need for an update.

Although consumers may not appreciate the technical aspects of health care, the public does have strong opinions about what constitutes a safe health care experience. The consumer's view of health services safety is covered in chapter 1. Comments obtained through interviews with patients, family members, and health care professionals illustrate the value of involving consumers in the patient safety movement. The greatest challenge may be achieving a culture of safety that welcomes patient involvement. Many health care professionals subscribe to a "culture of individual accountability" that can inhibit collaboration with patients and their family members. If active consumer involvement is one key to improving safety, practitioners must change their beliefs. Health care is so complex that every member of the health care team, including the patient, must play a role in preventing mistakes.

Physicians who believe that safety depends primarily on the actions of health care practitioners may not readily perceive opportunities for patients to improve health care services. Physicians' beliefs about individual accountability are shaped during education and training and reinforced by the fault-based medical liability system. In chapter 2, Dr. Joel Mattison, a plastic and reconstructive surgeon, describes how the classic medical model has suppressed the voice of health care consumers and why changes in the traditional patient-physician relationship are needed to improve patient safety. Dr. Mattison contends that patients can be involved in the safety movement if they are just given the correct information and the right tools for the job. Practitioners and organizations committed to patient-centered care have for years sought to empower patients and family members to speak up and work collaboratively with the health care team. Only recently have these efforts incorporated safety improvement strategies.

Swain and Spath, authors of chapter 3, assert that engaging consumers in health care safety requires health care professionals to first understand how things look from the patient's perspective. A real-life case study illustrates why patients want to be treated like responsible adults capable of assimilating information, asking informed questions, and having reasonable expectations. Results from recent studies of patient involvement in safety are detailed in this chapter—providing further proof that consumers can take an active role as safety partners if caregivers provide a supportive environment. Chapter 3 contains numerous strategies and techniques that can be used to teach patients how to stay safe as they navigate the confusing, and sometimes treacherous, health care system. Some of these strategies are from forward-thinking organizations that have advanced beyond mere information sharing.

Involving consumers in health care safety improvement is the right thing to do; however, practitioners may find it challenging to engage patients and family members in error prevention activities. Some patients may legitimately choose not to be involved. Often, practitioners may need to overcome communication or cultural barriers. Impediments to effective patient-practitioner collaboration can also originate from the attitudes and actions of health care professionals themselves. In chapter 4, the common collaboration obstacles on both sides of the patient-practitioner partnership are described by Pelling, along with strategies for surmounting these hurdles.

Health literacy—the consumer's ability to understand and act on printed or verbal health information—affects all aspects of health care, including patient safety. Patients or family members lacking sufficient health literacy are less able to effectively partner with caregivers. In chapter 5, nationally recognized health literacy experts Garcia and Brach describe the impact of low health literacy on safety partnerships and offer recommendations on how caregivers can overcome this barrier.

One of the most significant obstacles to an effective patient partnership is the health care professional's perceived threat of legal actions. Physicians, nurses, and other caregivers may be reluctant to engage patients as partners in preventing errors if such interactions will increase the risk of liability lawsuits. In chapter 6, two health law specialists, Saxton and Finkelstein, suggest that many of the liability fears associated with open and honest practitioner-patient dialogue are overstated. These attorneys describe the legal, cultural, and regulatory issues affecting information sharing and disclosure and offer suggestions for overcoming many of the perceived legal barriers.

Just a few years ago it would have been unheard of for a health care organization to invite a patient or family member to be part of the investigation of an adverse event. Yet some forward-thinking organizations are doing just that. Zimmerman and Amori, authors of chapter 7, describe how patient-centered care and transparency can mend potentially adversarial relationships between patients and providers. The authors suggest that one way of regaining this trust is by involving patients or family members in safety improvement evaluations—including sentinel event investigations. In this chapter, the potential legal implications are covered as well as what to consider when inviting patients or family members to participate on safety improvement task groups with physicians and staff members.

Involving patients in the safety movement will require a concerted effort on the part of health leaders to create an environment that embraces patients as partners in service delivery. In chapter 8, Dr. Thomas Royer details his involvement in the organization-wide patient safety efforts at the more than thirty hospitals, long-term care centers, physician offices, and outpatient clinics comprising CHRISTUS Health. As president and CEO of CHRISTUS Health, Dr. Royer is committed to gaining the trust and confidence of customers through reduction of errors, as well as through patient-centered care strategies.

Royal Oak Beaumont Hospital in Royal Oak, Michigan, is one of several forward-thinking health care organizations committed to involving consumers in medical error prevention. In chapter 9, Beauregard and Dr. Winokur describe how the organization is putting the patient into patient safety by creating a supportive culture and providing opportunities for education and partnership. The team at the hospital has created a firm foundation of patient safety that allows for ever-expanding involvement of patients and their families. In this chapter, readers learn more about how the organization is strengthening this involvement.

Thankfully, we are past the tipping point when it comes to involving patients and family members in our safety initiatives. Most agree that creating safety partnerships with consumers is the right thing to do. However, we still have many untapped opportunities and much to learn. As I said in the preface to *Partnering with Patients to Reduce Medical Errors*, this is not going to be easy. Yet, just as in 2003, I firmly believe that the end result is worth the effort. We'll have a safer health care system in which all members of the health care team, including patients, communicate effectively and support one another in achieving the best possible outcomes.

Patrice L. Spath
Forest Grove, Oregon
November 2007

Acknowledgments

I am pleased to express my appreciation of the many contributions of health care organizations and professionals dedicated to involving patients and family members in safety initiatives. This book would not have been possible without their unwavering commitment to safety partnerships and high-quality patient care.

Engaging Patients
as Safety Partners

1

Safety from the Patient's Point of View

Patrice L. Spath, BA, RHIT

Consumer safety is big business in the United States. Numerous national and state regulatory agencies and independent oversight bodies watch over the quality of products and services in an effort to ensure that consumers are protected from economic and/or physical harm. Consumer advocacy groups alert government regulators to new safety problems or dangerous products that have evaded the current systems of inspection or sanction. Consumer associations and lawyers (joined by an alliance of lawyers and politicians) often help to bring about new consumer protection laws. Professional organizations offer another layer of safety protection for consumers through the development of licensure or certification requirements, professional standards, and self-governance. All of these groups carry out the more general role of information sharing and consumer education.

Consumer materials generally fall into one of three broad categories: education, information, or promotion. Education materials are designed to help consumers understand key safety issues about a product or service. Information materials generally focus on providing safety tips, checklists, and other aids to help individuals stay safe when using a particular product or service. Promotion materials are designed primarily to sell a product, service, or image, although they may also have an educational or informational aspect. Growth of the consumer movement in the 1960s and 1970s led to the introduction of hazard warnings on consumer products ranging from household chemical cleaners to food products to major appliances.

Similar cautionary warnings about consumer services soon became commonplace. Consumers were taught how to make safe choices when selecting home improvement contractors, financial investment counselors, and other service providers.

Health Care Consumer Protection

With the establishment of a competitive health care market in 1994 and the subsequent spread of managed care, consumers began to express concerns about the quality and safety of health care services. Groups such as the Consumer Coalition for Quality Health Care were formed for the purpose of ensuring that consumers had access to a health care system that provided meaningful consumer information and choice, consumer participation, and grievance and appeals rights for individuals denied coverage or services. Horror stories about "drive-thru" baby deliveries and other seemingly inappropriate cost-cutting measures led to an increasing public outcry about declining health care quality and safety. It was also during this time that consumers began to assume more personal ownership for health care quality.

The need for individual involvement in health care quality was reinforced by the Consumer Bill of Rights and Responsibilities issued in November 1997 by the President's Advisory Commission on Consumer Protection and Quality in the Health Care Industry.[1] In providing consumers with a set of rights and protections, the commission acknowledged that individual consumers must assume certain responsibilities. These responsibilities include playing an active role in the treatment and management of their health and asking questions of their health care providers. The commission also encouraged health care providers to communicate more clearly with patients and their families about diagnoses, treatment options, and treatment protocols.

Patient participation began with encouraging individuals to become involved in making decisions about their personal health care. It is now expanding to embrace patient and family involvement in error prevention. As this latter agenda is advanced throughout the health care industry, it is likely that some will question whether patients are capable of understanding and promoting safety and preventing errors. In other words, does the individual patient have a purposeful role in patient safety, or is the theory merely patient-centered rhetoric that will ultimately have little influence on health care safety? Health care is often technical and requires background knowledge of medicine to understand it. Consumers may misunderstand some health care processes or take information out of context. Patients can speak from their own experiences with health services, and this expertise can be valuable from the perspective of customer satisfaction. However, will embracing the patient as an active member of the health care team yield benefits in terms of patient safety?

To address this question, let's consider another situation in which consumers have limited ability to safeguard their personal safety. An analogy to the consumer's health care experience is airline travel. Passengers on an airplane have little control over the safety of the travel event. The average airline traveler does not have background knowledge of aeronautics, nor does the traveler understand the mechanical workings of an airplane. It is unlikely the typical airplane passenger would be able to recognize or prevent the usual causes of airline accidents.[2] Yet the airline industry has acknowledged that safe air travel is a shared responsibility. Government regulators, manufacturers, members of the airline industry, and passengers are all viewed as playing a role in air safety. The following are some strategies, suggested by the Boeing Company, that airline travelers can use to protect themselves from being injured by the effects of turbulence:

- Always wear your seat belt when seated.
- Hold on to the seat backs or overhead bins when walking in the cabin.

- Listen to all safety announcements and follow flight crew instructions.
- Be careful when opening overhead bins following turbulence.[3]

An airplane passenger doesn't have to know how to construct an airplane or use navigational equipment to be an active participant in preventing injuries during severe turbulence. If explained in layperson terms, travelers can even figure out some of the "unknowns" of airline travel, such as what all the noises represent and what actions the pilots are accomplishing during the flight. Passengers are considered partners in air safety, and for this reason preflight and in-flight announcements to engage passengers in this role of partner are mandatory.

Consumer Involvement—Gaining Ground

Why haven't health care consumers been embraced as partners in safety as they have in other industries? Some speculate it is because health professionals have been reluctant to admit that mistakes happen; yet it is doubtful that members of other industries are any more willing to own up to errors. It is more likely that consumers have not been invited to be partners in health care safety because no one ever thought to ask. The public has customarily relied on government regulators and members of the health care industry to protect the quality and safety of health care services. The classic advice to medical professionals, *Primum non nocere* (First, do no harm), implies that the action and decision making rest in the hands of the physician, with no role for the patient.[4] Why would consumers feel the need to be involved in medical error prevention when practitioners promise not to knowingly harm patients and government regulators (and attorneys) punish the people or organizations that fail to live up to this promise?

What's been missing in health care are routine "preflight" and "in-flight" safety announcements—consumers have thus not felt the need or desire to be actively engaged in the safety movement. Patients are now beginning to understand that they play a role in keeping themselves safe during the health care experience. A patient focus has always underpinned medical professional rhetoric but has had surprisingly little influence on the development of true patient-practitioner partnerships. With the quality and safety of health care perceived to be inadequate on many counts, the traditional passive role of consumers is being scrutinized and questioned by the public as well as those in the health care industry.

In the 2001 Institute of Medicine report *Crossing the Quality Chasm*, patient-centeredness was recognized as an essential component of quality care.[5] *Patient-centeredness* was described as including both the patient's experience of care and the presence of an effective partnership between clinician and patient (and the patient's family, when appropriate). Patient-centeredness as a safety improvement strategy provided the impetus for the national "Speak Up" campaign advocated by the Joint Commission in March 2002[6] and similar consumer outreach initiatives by the Agency for Healthcare Research and Quality[7] and others. At the start of these campaigns, there was only anecdotal evidence that actively involved patients could have an effect on safety. Lacking such research, many groups were unwilling at that time to endorse patient involvement as a worthwhile safety intervention. None of the thirty safe practice recommendations found in the 2003 National Quality Forum (NQF) report *Safe Practices for Better Healthcare: A Consensus Report*[8] explicitly addressed patient involvement. However, the NQF acknowledged that patients want to take a more active role in reducing their chance of experiencing a medical error. For this reason, the NQF recommended more research to determine the efficacy of patient involvement as a safety improvement strategy—Can patients recognize potential errors? Will patients be willing and able to participate in error prevention strategies? Will their involvement actually reduce errors? The NQF recommendation, as well as proposals in earlier work funded by the Agency for Healthcare Research and Quality,[9] spawned several research studies. Some of these noteworthy study findings are summarized in table 1-1.

Table 1-1. Summary of Studies Evaluating the Efficacy of Patient Involvement as a Safety Improvement Strategy

Question	Study (Year)	Findings/Conclusions
Can patients recognize potential errors?	Kuzel et al. (2004)[1]	Patients were able to identify problematic ambulatory care incidents, many which were linked to specific harms. The incidents included errors of omission and commission and occurred in all phases of primary care.
	Weingart et al. (2005)[2]	Patients were able retrospectively to identify "problems," "mistakes," and "injuries" that occurred during hospitalization. Many of these patient-identified events were not captured by the hospital incident reporting system or recorded in the medical record.
Will patients be willing and able to participate in error prevention strategies?	Weingart et al. (2004)[3]	Medical inpatients (or their surrogates) were willing to participate in an intervention designed to decrease adverse drug events. Caregivers found the intervention unobtrusive and beneficial at reducing medication errors. However, patients had a limited capacity to partner with clinicians due to the acuity or severity of their illness or cognitive impairment. Interventions that rely on patient and family participation may be more effective in populations with few comorbid illnesses (e.g., labor and delivery, elective surgery), with reliable family involvement (e.g., pediatrics), and with satisfactory functional status (e.g., ambulatory care).
	Entwistle, Mello, and Brennan (2005)[4]	Consumers should be involved in developing safety advisory materials. Distributing safety advisories to patients may not be sufficient to create partnerships; *active* encouragement and a supportive environment is needed. Rather than rely on patients to remember to act, systems should be designed to enable people to contribute appropriately by default.

Table 1-1. (Continued)

Question	Study (Year)	Findings/Conclusions
Will patients be willing and able to participate in error prevention strategies?	Hibbard et al. (2005)[5]	Engaging patients in safety requires the use of language that is understandable and compelling. *Medical errors* is a more effective phrase than *patient safety* for communicating with the public. To have maximum impact, educational approaches to engage patients should aim to increase both the patients' sense of self-efficacy and understanding of the effectiveness of the recommended actions.
	Waterman et al. (2006)[6]	Patients are generally comfortable with error prevention; however, participation varies according to how comfortable they are with the recommended actions. For example, many feel comfortable asking about the purpose of their medication, whereas they are less comfortable questioning caregivers about hand-washing practices. Educational interventions to increase patients' comfort with error prevention will be necessary to help them become more engaged.
	Peters et al. (2006)[7]	How much consumers worry about the possibility of a medical error is a strong predictor of whether they will take precautionary actions to prevent errors. An understanding of how worry influences patients' preventive efforts will help in building communication strategies that will effectively engage them as vigilant partners in care.
Will patient involvement actually reduce errors?	Weingart et al. (2004)[3]	Hospital nurses anecdotally reported that medication errors had been prevented because a medical inpatient or family member identified drug-related problems.

(Continued on next page)

Table 1-1. (Continued)

Question	Study (Year)	Findings/Conclusions
Will patient involvement actually reduce errors?	Pames et al. (2007)[8]	Ambulatory providers reported that in some situations it was patient vigilance (asking questions, seeking solutions) that prevented harm which could have resulted from a medical error.

[1] A. J. Kuzel, S. H. Woolf, V. J. Gilchrist, J. D. Engel, T. A. LaVeist, C. Vincent, and R. M. Frankel, "Patient Reports of Preventable Problems and Harms in Primary Health Care," *Annals of Family Medicine* 2, no. 4 (2004): 333–40.

[2] S. N. Weingart, O. Pagovich, D. Z. Sands, J. M. Li, M. D. Aronson, R. B. Davis, D. W. Bates, and R. S. Phillips, "What Can Hospitalized Patients Tell Us about Adverse Events? Learning from Patient-Reported Incidents," *Journal of General Internal Medicine* 20, no. 9 (2005): 830–36.

[3] S. N. Weingart, M. Toth, J. Eneman, M. D. Aronson, D. Z. Sands, A. N. Ship, R. B. Davis, and R. S. Phillips, "Lessons from a Patient Partnership Intervention to Prevent Adverse Drug Events," *International Journal for Quality in Health Care* 16, no. 6 (2004): 499–507.

[4] V. A. Entwistle, M. M. Mello, and T. A. Brennan, "Advising Patients about Patient Safety: Current Initiatives Risk Shifting Responsibility," *Joint Commission Journal on Quality and Patient Safety* 31, no. 9 (2005): 483–94.

[5] J. H. Hibbard, E. Peters, P. Slovic, and M. Tusler, "Can Patients Be Part of the Solution? Views on Their Role in Preventing Medical Errors," *Medical Care Research* 62, no. 5 (2005): 601–16.

[6] A. D. Waterman, T. H. Gallagher, J. Garbutt, B. M. Waterman, V. Fraser, and T. E. Burroughs, "Brief Report: Hospitalized Patients' Attitudes about and Participation in Error Prevention," *Journal of General Internal Medicine* 21, no. 4 (2006): 367–70.

[7] E. Peters, P. Slovic, J. H. Hibbard, and M. Tusler, "Why Worry? Worry, Risk Perceptions, and Willingness to Act to Reduce Medical Errors," *Health Psychology* 25, no. 2 (2006): 144–52.

[8] B. Pames, D. Fernald, J. Quintela, R. Araya-Guerra, J. Wesfall, D. Harris, and W. Pace, "Stopping the Error Cascade: A Report on Ameliorators," *Quality and Safety in Health Care* 16, no. 1 (2007): 12–16.

Research generally supports the notion that patients can recognize errors or problematic situations. If adequately educated and provided a supportive environment, patients and family members may be willing and able to partner with caregivers to prevent errors or mitigate harmful error effects. Patient involvement could result in a safer health care experience as suggested by anecdotal findings in research studies, incident analyses in patient safety literature, and public media reports.[10,11,12]

In 2006, the NQF updated its list of safe practices, and in the new edition it recommended development of strategies to involve consumers in the implementation of safe practices.[13] In just a few short years the patient safety movement went from skepticism about the value of patient involvement to a realization that patient-centeredness can be an important contributor to reducing error-related harm. Like the airline industry, where passengers have a role to play in safe air travel, the health care industry has come to view safe health care as a shared opportunity with patients. Our next challenge is learning how to facilitate patient involvement in a practical and engaging manner.

Health care consumers are similar to airline passengers in that they have a limited technical understanding of the health care experience. But health care consumers, like airline passengers, can become knowledgeable safety partners. Patients and their families will choose to be involved in different ways and at different degrees of intensity. Just as some airline passengers don't perform their safety duties, some patients will remain passive and expect health care professionals to assume all accident prevention responsibilities. Patients with chronic illnesses (like frequent air travelers) may wish to become exceptionally skilled at controlling the health care experience in an effort to reduce the risk of personal harm. All health care professionals should be striving toward developing a variety of interventions and methods that allow every consumer an opportunity to participate in the patient safety movement in a way that suits her or his needs and level of commitment.

Changing the Patient-Practitioner Relationship

Many patients are keen to take some responsibility for optimizing the outcomes of the health care experience.[14] Allowing patients to fulfill this role to their satisfaction, however, will require a change in the social relationship between health care professionals and patients. Figure 1-1 illustrates the characteristics of the traditional paternalistic health care professional and the traits that must be adopted if patient-practitioner collaboration is to be fully realized.

Hospital organizations that are forming safety partnerships with patients and their families readily acknowledge the need for a profound cultural shift. In the words of Judith Napier, MSN, co-chair of the Patient Safety Committee at Children's Hospitals and Clinics of Minnesota, "Optimizing patient care requires creating an institutional expectation, a shared belief, that patient safety is everyone's responsibility."[15] The need for a culture change in health care is reinforced in the report *Collaborative Education to Ensure Patient Safety*, jointly published by the Council on Graduate Medical Education (COGME) and the National Advisory Council on Nurse Education and Practice (NACNEP). One of the major recommendations in the COGME-NACNEP report is that patient safety will require a significant change in the cultures that guide current medicine and nursing practices. The councils recognize that physicians and nurses will have to adjust their own practice approaches to encourage patients to become educated and to participate in their own health care.[16]

Figure 1-1. Old and New Concepts of the Professional Role

The Paternalistic Professional	The Collaborative Professional
• Master of knowledge and skills	• Shared learning
• Unilateral ownership of quality and safety (patient is dependent)	• Interdependent relationship (patient is empowered)
• Individual accountability	• Collective responsibility
• Detached	• Engaged

The education of health care professionals, regulation and other forms of accountability, decision making, reward systems, performance measurement, and even the very nature of patient autonomy and involvement must be rethought. Useful as it might be, inviting patients to be partners in the safety movement will amount to little more than tinkering with the old model of health care unless there are reforms in education, regulation, professionalism, and the other health care subsystems that influence quality.

What Consumers Have to Offer

The limited availability of physicians in the first third of the nineteenth century prompted many Americans to depend on self-care to treat recurrent illnesses. There was also a far-reaching distrust of physicians, whose painful treatments included bloodletting and violent purgatives.[17] Eventually, medical practices changed, and physicians and other health professionals became more available. Somewhere in this evolution, the patient's self-responsibility for health services, as well as the voice of the health care customer, got lost. Health care became something that was done to—not with—patients.

In the early 1990s, the public's trust in the health care industry began to erode again. Several factors contributed to this mistrust, including the public perception that the industry failed in self-regulation and that health care organizations were putting their own interests above those of patients and the public.[18] The well-publicized reports of unpleasant outcomes resulting from medical errors caused even further mistrust. This general mistrust persists in spite of more rigorous regulatory oversight and nationwide patient safety improvement initiatives.

With lessening confidence in the quality and safety of health services, consumers are becoming self-advocates. The regular exercise of self-advocacy has led to more discerning health care consumers, many of whom are alert to quality problems and eager to contribute to the patient safety movement.

Can Consumers Distinguish Safe Care?

The consumer's perception of health service safety is based on input from a variety of sources: personal experiences, others' personal experiences (including general beliefs handed down through generations), and the media (books, movies, documentaries, advertisements, and news—factual and fictitious, positive and negative). Of course, the perceptions of patients or their caregivers may be inaccurate, but perception is patients' reality and will definitely influence beliefs.

The consumer's judgment about the safety of a particular health care experience is also influenced by factors more subtle than perceptions, such as the neatness of the surroundings, the practitioner's demeanor, or whether caregivers appear confident. Again, the patient or caregiver may be right or very misinformed, but when health services are needed and a decision must be made, people will use whatever information they have available. Because the consumer's assessment of patient safety is based on several factors, the same health care experience may be considered unsafe by one person and safe by another.

If consumers are to be embraced as active partners in the patient safety movement, health care professionals cannot hold to the premise that the public is not in a position to understand or judge the safety of health services. Active participation implies the sharing of information and opinions, joint problem solving, and joint responsibility. Another factor influencing consumers' opinions about the safety of health services is their understanding or belief that the health care organization is committed to providing safe health services. Unless they have some reason to believe this commitment exists, they may suspect otherwise. Listening to and acting on the safety concerns of consumers can go a long way toward demonstrating a provider's dedication to patient safety.

In preparation for the writing of this chapter, a number of health care consumers (patients and caregivers) were interviewed to determine their understanding of safe health care practices and what makes them feel unsafe. Some of the people surveyed have little or no medical expertise, whereas others currently work (or have worked) in the health care industry. The comments of these consumers are found in the next sections, together with some background information about the person offering the comments. The responses are not intended to represent a valid research study, nor are they an adequate sampling of all health care consumers. Respondents were self-selected from the larger group of people who were invited to participate. As such, these consumers may have stronger opinions or more to say about health care safety than the average person may. Even with these shortcomings, health care professionals are encouraged to take the comments to heart. All respondents have expertise based on their lived experience of illness and health services. The value of listening to and acting on the comments of these consumers is best summed up in the words of Norman McLean in his book *A River Runs Through It* (University of Chicago Press, 1989): "All there is to thinking is seeing something noticeable which makes you see something you weren't noticing which makes you see something that isn't even visible."

Views on Safety from Patients

People who have been recipients of health services were asked to respond to the following question: What would a safe health experience look and feel like to you? The responses were influenced by several factors, including the person's age, health status, personal experiences, and convictions. To aid in interpreting the respondents' comments, some background information is provided.

Male, 49 years old, Alabama. Background: Educator in allied health professional degree program (nonclinical). Regular user of health care services as the result of a variety of chronic conditions.

Overall, a safe health experience would be one that has no negative outcomes—no mishaps, no adverse reactions to treatment or medication, no unintended harm to the patient. I would feel safe if all information regarding my previous care was always available in my chart along with my allergies, and so on. The treating physicians and nurses should understand the medications that I am on and the potential for any adverse reactions with any additionally prescribed medications. Feeling safe also means to me that I am receiving the appropriate treatment for my condition and that I am able to freely discuss the treatment being given.

Female, 47 years old, Colorado. Background: Patient advocate specializing in support services for those injured by medical errors. She describes herself as "basically a healthy person with only periodic visits to the doctor."

In order to make health care experiences safer for all concerned, there has to be communication between the doctor, the staff, and the patient. When my husband was in the hospital, his primary care physician did not see him once. It took at least three calls for the doctor to even call me back, and the urologist who did the original biopsy did not call back even after repeated calls. Let's just say this did not inspire confidence in the doctors.

Patients must be ready and willing to assume some responsibility for their medical care. They must come into the office with a list of medications they are taking and ask questions about interactions. Maybe they need to ask these questions of their druggist or contact the manufacturer of the medication.

Male, 42 years old, Pennsylvania. Background: Editor for a health care magazine. No medical expertise or health care experience. He is in good health with only sporadic physician visits.

A safe health care experience to me would be one in which the staff asked me many questions and reassured me that no matter how many questions I asked, I was not bothering them. I want to know that I can ask any question I may have. Also, the staff would explain everything they were doing. For example, if they started examining my stomach, they would say, "I'm checking here because. . . ."

The safe health care experience would start at the point of making the appointment with a competent, professional scheduler who could at least understand my problem and treat it with the urgency required of the situation. If I stated that I was concerned about whatever condition I was calling about, and an appointment wasn't available for several weeks, I would expect the scheduler to tell me what options I had for being seen earlier, either by seeing another practitioner or being placed on a cancellation list.

Female, 41 years old, Georgia. Background: Product marketing manager for publishing firm. No medical expertise or health care experience. She is an average user of health care services with no chronic conditions.

My idea of a safe health care experience: Someone would call me a couple of days prior to my health service appointment to pre-register me, or I would be given a phone number or Web site where I can preregister. When presenting for the appointment, I would give my name, and the provider would already have all of the information necessary to care for me. The nurse would have preread my chart and know why I was there and would ask questions for clarification. If it were necessary for the practitioner to touch me, he or she would wash up in front of me so that I knew it was sanitary. The physician would spend a few minutes reading the nurses' notes and would be aware of my presenting problem before entering my room and would wash up in front of me before touching me. He would ask for clarification, examine me thoroughly, and allow time for me to ask questions and ask about treatment options. He would make a recommendation of what treatment plan he felt best but would include me in the decision-making process. If lab work or diagnostic tests were called for, the physician would make sure that I understood exactly what was going to be done and where and all of the potential side effects. The doctor would let me know if any follow-up is necessary and be specific about when I should make another appointment if one is needed.

For lab work or tests, the technicians would give a brief description of their understanding of the presenting problem and what diagnostic tests were to be performed. This would give me the opportunity to make sure that the tests being performed were the same as those the physician had told me about. The technicians would let me know how my tests and lab work were going to be processed so there was no chance that they would be misplaced or mislabeled as someone else's results. If possible, I would see my name and account number on the film, or tube, or whatever. At the conclusion of the test, I would be told when the results would be back and how to obtain them. If I were told that the doctor would contact me, then the doctor's office would call.

Anytime anyone was going to administer medication to me, he or she would state what the medication was, what it was for, and confirm that I was the person who was to receive the medication. If the person administering the medication had to touch me, he or she would wash his or her hands in front of me prior to doing so.

Female, 59 years old, New York. Background: Antique dealer and amateur artist. No medical expertise or any other health care background. She only occasionally sees a physician; however, a few years ago she cared for an elderly relative who had several chronic conditions and multiple hospital admissions.

Society has unrealistically high health care expectations. Not every injured, sick, or dying person will be healed, and medical accidents will happen because of human error. There must be an extensive campaign to modify the public's unrealistic expectations. If my expectations are more in line with reality, then it will be easier for me to have the perception of a safe health care experience.

In a safe health care experience, a team of health care professionals is responsible for my care. They understand that I am also a member of the team. Members of the team are accessible to me. Information is shared with me. I have input with regard to their plans for my care. Because we communicate and I am part of the process, I am not a helpless victim. I would also feel safer if I had a patient advocate to watch over my care when I'm not able to personally keep track of what's happening. Every patient needs an advocate.

Ideally, my medical history and medications are part of a centralized database of patient information that is easily accessible to my team. The team responsible for my care is not sleep deprived. If they work long hours without sufficient rest, their decision-making abilities could be impaired and my safety will be jeopardized.

Male, 59 years old, South Carolina. Background: Higher education professor and education design specialist. He is a member of a hospital governing board.

I would feel safe if I received a quality diagnosis that was offered by a reputable professional and concurred with by at least two or three other professional opinions. My health care providers would need to be fully certified or accredited and technically proficient. Staff caring for me should take the time to explain and respond to my concerns and be spiritually enlightened. My surroundings should be aesthetically pleasing, and my family members and other significant individuals (clergy, attorney) should have appropriate access to me.

The last consideration in my safety would be adequate follow-up procedures. This would include timely and routine checks on my progress. Also, I should be provided an opportunity to give feedback to my providers and be encouraged to make suggestions for improving health care services.

Male, 56 years old, Georgia. Background: Health care journalist; no clinical background. He has type 2 diabetes requiring periodic outpatient visits.

Every medical experience I have is colored by the fact that I have type 2 diabetes. Accordingly, the first thing that would make me feel safe with health care professionals would be the fact that they knew my history and that they were well versed in all aspects of the disease. I would expect to be asked what my latest blood sugars are, how I am feeling, and what I am doing in terms of diet and exercise. My physical examination should include tests specifically designed to assess possible complications from diabetes (retinopathy, circulation problems, etc.).

I feel safe with a health care provider when he or she seems genuinely concerned about my well-being and willing to listen to me and answer my questions. I also feel safe with an individual who seems confident, knowledgeable, and honest about the possible side effects of any drugs I may need to take or any procedure about to occur. Honesty, openness, caring, concern, and knowledge—these are what inspire my confidence and make me feel safe.

Views on Safety from Caregivers

It has been estimated that more than 50 million people in the United States provide care for a chronically ill, disabled, or aged family member or friend during any given year.[19] Many caregivers provide full-time care for a family member or friend and deal with a wide array of medical conditions and diagnoses. The caregiver's perception of health care safety is significantly influenced by the experiences shared with his or her spouse, parent, children, sibling, or friend. People serving as caregivers offer a perspective on safety that is different from that of the patient. To gain the caregiver's point of view for this chapter, members of the National Family Caregivers Association were invited to respond to the question, What would a safe health experience for your loved one look and feel like to you?

Female, 45 years old, Texas. Background: Caregiver for her husband, who suffered a stroke and kidney failure about ten years ago. She has a degree in chemistry and biology but has not worked in the health care industry.

Here are my suggestions for making the health care experience safer for patients:

1. Chairs (dialysis chairs, wheelchairs, and so on) and stretchers used for patients who may be physically incapacitated should always have locks on the wheels and should always be locked for patient transfer.

2. Staff should always communicate with patients and/or their family members as to the patient's abilities, discomforts, aches, and disabilities before moving them. They should continue to check on the patient's level of comfort as they proceed.

3. Contact information should be posted prominently so that patients, family members, and even employees can easily inform the appropriate building personnel of safety concerns.

4. Listen to the concerns of patients and their family members. Physicians and other staff should appreciate that when patients or family members bring up safety concerns, they view the issues as real problems and are only trying to help the professionals do their job better and keep themselves or their loved ones safe.

5. Physicians and other staff should understand that when patients or family members request certain medications, tests, or other treatments, they often know what they are talking about. A physician or nurse who may have only just met the patient can't know as much as the patient who has the chronic condition or a family member who has been caring for that person.

6. Most of all, health care professionals should remember that they are human and will make mistakes. There is no harm in checking with the patient or family members for a second opinion. And there is no excuse for ignoring or trivializing patient input. Emotional security is just as important to the patient as physical safety.

7. Last, staff members should also keep in mind that patients are human. They are not machines or slabs of meat to throw on a table to poke and prod. Patients are not insignificant; they are human beings who need your help.

Female, 41 years old, New Jersey. Background: Caregiver for her 11-year-old daughter who has multiple chronic conditions, including kidney disease (renal agenesis, renal dysplasia, Grade IV bilateral vesicoureteral reflux), and autism (Asperger syndrome).

A "safe experience" would be one in which I know a procedure is being done properly with no hesitation on the part of the professional and minimal discomfort for my child. That said, I think that family caregivers need to be present at all times, educated about medical procedures, and be vigilant observers. I've had a few instances where errors occurred even in my presence:

- A pediatric nurse tried to use an adult-size catheter on my infant daughter. I stopped her. I happened to know it was the adult size because I had been hospitalized during my pregnancy and was catheterized several times. I called a doctor in to perform the procedure.
- The laboratory did not check my daughter's immunization records and gave her an extra hepatitis B shot. The error wasn't noticed until I pointed out on the chart that she had already received three shots. If they'd had me sign a consent form (as was usual), the mistake might have been noticed before the injection was given. My daughter is a medically fragile child who previously went into shock after a DPT immunization.
- During an MRI, the portion of my daughter's spine being checked for tethered cord due to spina bifida occulta was not well supported as she was coming out of anesthesia.
- While my daughter was under anesthesia for the MRI, no one even thought to put a pull-up diaper on her, so I had to do it. She has enuresis due to her kidney disease.

Views on Safety from Health Care Professionals

Although patient safety is a shared commitment among all health care professionals, many professionals are not certain of how to go about effectively involving consumers in the safety movement. Practitioners' training and work experiences significantly influence their patient safety beliefs. To broaden the views of health care professionals, a physician and nurse were asked to respond to the question, What would the health care experience be like if patients and families were actively involved in making health care safer?

Male, pediatrician, Ohio. Background: After retiring from an active practice, he worked as vice president for medical affairs in two hospitals and as a part-time medical director for a health plan. At the present time, he consults with several health care organizations to address such issues as Joint Commission and regulatory compliance, physician practice management, medical staff administration and reorganization, and physician education in medical staff functions and responsibilities.

A safe health care experience is one in which there is effective communication between patients and physicians. Unfortunately, for the most part, physician-patient contact has yet to become a true interactive exchange of information with both parties striving to reach a mutually satisfactory care goal. Physicians, by training or because of perceived time constraints, frequently present a closed attitude to patients. Sensing this, patients are often intimidated from actively participating in their care. When patients are passive participants, they don't volunteer information and refrain from asking questions. In this circumstance, neither the physician nor the patient receives the information and understanding necessary for a safe health care experience.

Physicians have to accept that patients come armed with more information from outside, albeit not necessarily always reliable, sources. Patients want to discuss that information with the physician. Physicians must take the lead in presenting an environment where the patient feels free to exchange information and cooperate with, or challenge, the diagnostic plan or the course of treatment. The physician's people skills have to be honed to match his or her technical skills.

To create a more satisfying patient-practitioner relationship, physicians must allow interchange to occur and must respect the patient's desire and right to question and challenge. It must come to be accepted that this type of relationship is not, by definition, confrontational. The increasing complexity of patient care demands this type of patient-physician interaction. When patients have a better understanding of their condition and treatment, they can become the first line of defense against misadventures and unsafe situations.

Female, registered nurse, California. Background: She has twenty-five years of health care experience as a critical care nurse and a certified health care quality professional. For the past eight years she has been on the "patient side" of health care, having suffered a spinal cord injury, which resulted in quadriplegia. Two years after her injury, she was diagnosed with breast cancer. She describes herself as "an experienced inpatient," having had three hospitalizations for a total of four weeks, two months in acute rehab, and four surgical procedures.

Patients are much more likely to perceive their health care experience as safe when they are included as active participants rather than treated as helpless victims. Patients should be encouraged to participate as fully as possible in their care. From my perspective as both a nurse and a patient, the following suggestions are offered to physicians, nurses, and other health care professionals:

- Actively listen to your patients' questions, concerns, and observations. As a patient, I feel safer when I perceive staff to be listening to me.
- Encourage patients to ask questions or provide input to their care whenever you are with them for whatever reason. Patients don't feel safe if the only way they can get the caregiver's attention is by using their call light or lodging a complaint.
- Teach those patients who are coherent and interested everything that is reasonable for them to know. Teaching should be done verbally with the same instructions and information provided in writing.
- Encourage your patients to notify you or another staff member if they believe something is "not right" or "abnormal."
- Teach those patients with an expressed desire to know (just ask first) how to be observant for problems and when to call for assistance (for example, IV line or injection site concerns, what the alarms mean, what should occur when an IV bottle is empty, when to be concerned about a dressing, and so on).
- Give a medication sheet to coherent hospitalized patients and cross-check the medications with the patients before administration (including IVs). This collaboration is also a good time to teach safe medication administration practices to patients.

Provide patients with brief written descriptions of any new medications, similar to the instruction sheets that outpatient pharmacies provide to customers.

- Tell patients about the hand-washing policy. Ask them to speak up if practitioners entering the room fail to wash their hands before touching them.
- Provide mechanisms for your patients to share suggestions for improving the overall health care experience (ways to do things that are safer, smarter, quicker, and less costly) and ideas for making their own care better. When patients are able to share their views, they are more likely to be satisfied, and a satisfied patient feels safer.

The caveat to these recommendations is that communication must be free flowing and two way. Caregivers must establish relationships with their patients, even if very short term, and must be good listeners. In a safe environment, caregivers are confident, competent, communicative, and comfortable with their patients. They listen to their patients' concerns and ideas with sincere interest and then do what they say they will do to follow through. This may involve further communications with the patient, communications with other health care professionals, timely intervention, documentation, or reporting. To me, this makes for the best "feel safe" care.

Implications for Patient Safety

As the role of the health care consumer in patient safety receives increased attention, it is important to consider the opinions and preferences of patients and their families. Several primary themes can be found in the comments of those people participating in the formal interviews. Consumers want practitioners to treat patients with care, compassion, and honesty. They want practitioners to have a broader understanding of patients, one that takes into consideration the emotional, social, mental, spiritual, and physical dimensions of the person's medical condition. Patients want to be listened to and respected for their opinions. Patients, caregivers, and practitioners alike emphasized the importance of involving patients as part of the care team and teaching them what they can do to keep themselves safe. Despite the limitations of this informal survey process, the results are consistent with the study results summarized in table 1-1 above.

Francine R. Gaillour, MD, speculates that the trend toward active patient participation could lead to the emergence of a new medical specialty: the patient advocate.[20] According to Dr. Gaillour, the physician serving as a patient advocate would not provide any direct care; rather, he or she would play the role of translator of medical knowledge and facilitator of treatment decision making, helping the client sort through diagnosis, treatment, and care options. A patient advocate role, whether assumed by a physician, nurse, or other knowledgeable health care professional or layperson, could improve patient safety. For this reason, the National Patient Safety Foundation (NPSF) is committed to educating people about how a patient advocate can help health care safety. The NPSF brochure, "The Role of the Patient Advocate," offers tips for patients in choosing an advocate to look out for their best health care interests.[21]

Learning about Safety from Patients

Health care professionals are learning to value the expertise of patients, and many are eager to tap into a patient's experience to learn what can be done to improve the safety of health care. The National Patient Safety Agency (NPSA) in the United Kingdom is actively involving patients in several health service safety initiatives. In late 2002, the NPSA initiated a study to determine the root causes of problems surrounding the use of infusion devices to deliver fluids and drugs to patients. The NPSA researchers reviewed the global evidence on infusion device user errors; looked at best practices already taking place in the National Health Services; sought feedback from health professionals; and interviewed patients who had used a pump in the hospital for chemotherapy, pain control, or insulin control. The patient interviews elicited a great deal of information on what being on a pump feels like from the patient's viewpoint as well as many valid safety concerns. Study findings that concentrate on safety issues relevant to nurses and nursing care are presented in the appendix at the end of this chapter.[22]

In the United States, an increasing number of health care organizations are partnering with patients and families to create safer systems.[23] A pioneer in this effort is the Dana-Farber Cancer Institute (DFCI) in Boston. This facility sponsors both adult and pediatric patient/family advisory councils that are actively involved in the design, implementation, and assessment of safety initiatives and care overall. The co-chairs of the adult advisory committee attend meetings of DFCI's Adult Oncology Clinical Services Committee, where they participate in problem-solving discussions of patient safety–related concerns.[24] Children's Hospitals and Clinics of Minnesota has a family advisory council aimed at involving families in similar advisory roles.[25] The list of health care organizations reaching out to patients, family members, and the community to become involved in patient safety improvement efforts continues to grow.

Involving Patients on the Health Care Team

Safety is a system property that has yet to be achieved in health care. A safe system is one in which the entire health care system is designed to prevent errors and minimize the effects of ordinary human mistakes. By involving the patient as a member of the health care team, several pairs of eyes, each with a different perspective, can help make the system of care safer. Different members of the team may see red flags or opportunities at times and places that no single member of the team is in a position to see. A certain amount of good redundancy is built into the system when everyone is on the alert for mistakes. Health care processes must be made transparent so that everyone (including the patient) knows what is going on and why. Health care is so complex that no single discipline or care recipient can possibly maintain the situational awareness needed to prevent adverse events.

Nothing less than a revolution in medical culture may be needed to fully accept patients as legitimate members of the health care team. During his training, Dr. Marc Ringel sensed he was being constantly indoctrinated with two principles:

1. The doctor must know everything. It is not okay to say, "I don't know."
2. The doctor is to be in charge in every patient care situation. Everyone else, no matter what the expertise or knowledge of the patient, must defer to the physician.[26]

Only recently have medical schools begun to teach their students to be team players in the health care setting. Similar team training is advocated for other health care professionals.[27] Clearly, teaching health professionals to act as a team must be accomplished, or practitioners may never be able to fully embrace the patient as a valued team member. Although consumers may be positioned to bring about some improvements in the safety of health services, they cannot influence the curricula for doctors, nurses, and allied health professionals. It will be up to the academic community to fully adopt the 1998 recommendations of the Pew Commission, which urged education systems to ensure that graduates are successful in meeting the expectations of health care consumers.[28]

Patients don't want to believe that physicians, nurses, or other health care professionals make mistakes, especially when it is a caregiver they know and trust. Yet there is a growing public realization that mistakes happen and that the patient (and family members or caregiver) can play a part in reducing the chance of a harmful accident. The role of patients in health care safety is not limited to providing practitioners with the information necessary to do their job. To achieve the full safety benefit from patient involvement, health care organizations must incorporate patient feedback into safety improvement initiatives, set up opportunities for dialogue between patients and health care professionals, and incorporate the patient perspective into initial training and continuing education programs for caregivers.

At the patient-practitioner level, patients must be respected for the knowledge they have. This means listening and responding to patients' questions, handling problems so they don't recur, sharing information that empowers patients to prevent errors, and actively encouraging patients to be partners with the health care team. If you remain skeptical about patients' desire and ability to join the team, reread the comments from patients, family members, and health care professionals found earlier in this chapter.

The degree of patient participation in the treatment process depends on patients' physical and mental condition, willingness, knowledge, and experience. Yet patients always have some role in achieving a satisfactory outcome by committing to treatment, becoming educated enough to participate in the healing process, and being cooperative and compliant during and after care delivery. To play even a minor role in the patient safety movement, consumers must be taught how to communicate effectively with health care practitioners.

Raising the safety performance of a complex system like health care means recognizing that it is the people on the front lines who have to make and sustain change. Safe results every time cannot be mandated by regulatory agencies or organizational leaders. Rather, the focus must be on building the capacity of each member of the health care team to identify problems and improve the system. Every member of the team, including the patient, must be empowered to speak up and work collaboratively.

References

1. Advisory Commission on Consumer Protection and Quality in the Health Care Industry, "Appendix A. Consumer Bill of Rights and Responsibilities," in *Quality First: Better Health Care for All Americans* (1998) [http://www.hcqualitycommission.gov/final/append_a.html]. Accessed October 2007.
2. Common causes of airplane accidents: (1) failure to adequately compensate for wind conditions during takeoff and climb out; (2) takeoff in wind conditions beyond the pilot's or airplane's capabilities; (3) engine failure or loss of power after takeoff; (4) failure to maintain

adequate airspeed during takeoff and climb out, resulting in a departure stall; (5) attempting takeoff with too strong a tailwind component; (6) failure to compensate for high-density altitude conditions or attempting takeoff in high-density altitude conditions beyond the airplane's capabilities; and (7) improper configuration of the aircraft for weight and flight conditions. From J. K. Boatman, "Plan the Takeoff—And Take Off According to the Plan," *AOPA Pilot* (June 2001).

3. The Boeing Company, "What Can Passengers Do—Enhancing Your Air Travel Safety" (Chicago: Boeing) [http://www.boeing.com/commercial/safety/pf/pf_passenger_role.html]. Accessed October 2007.

4. J. D. Shelton, "The Harm of 'First, Do No Harm,'" *Journal of the American Medical Association* 284, no. 21 (2000): 2687–88.

5. Institute of Medicine, Committee on Health Care in America, *Crossing the Quality Chasm: A New Health System for the 21st Century* (Washington, DC: National Academies Press, 2001).

6. Joint Commission, "Care Recipients Urged to 'Speak Up' for Safer Health Care," *Joint Commission Perspectives* 22, no. 5 (2002): 3.

7. Agency for Healthcare Research and Quality, "Consumers & Patients. (Rockville, MD: Agency for Healthcare Research and Quality) [http://www.ahrq.gov/consumer/]. Accessed October 2007.

8. National Quality Forum, *Safe Practices for Better Healthcare: Summary. A Consensus Report* (Rockville, MD: Agency for Healthcare Research and Quality, August 2003) [http://www.ahrq.gov/qual/nqfpract.htm]. Accessed October 2007.

9. Agency for Healthcare Research and Quality, *Making Health Care Safer: A Critical Analysis of Patient Safety Practices.* Evidence Report/Technology Assessment: Number 43. AHRQ Publication No. 01-E058 (Rockville, MD: Agency for Healthcare Research and Quality, July 2001) [http://www.ahrq.gov/clinic/ptsafety/]. Accessed October 2007.

10. Pennsylvania Patient Safety Authority, "When Patients Speak—Collaboration in Patient Safety," *Patient Safety Advisory* 2, no. 1 (2005): 1–4.

11. Institute for Safe Medication Practices, "An Inquisitive Patient Is a Safe Patient. Persistence Pays Off," *ISMP Safe Medicine* 5, no. 5 (2007) [http://www.ismp.org/Newsletters/consumer/Issues/20070709.asp]. Accessed October 2007.

12. Liz Szabo, "Patient, Protect Thyself," *USA Today*, February 5, 2007 [http://www.usatoday.com/news/health/2007-02-04-patient-safety_x.htm]. Accessed October 2007.

13. National Quality Forum, *Safe Practices for Better Healthcare—2006 Update: A Consensus Report* (Washington, DC: National Quality Forum, 2006) [http://www.qualityforum.org/pdf/reports/safe_practices/txsppublic.pdf]. Accessed October 2007.

14. D. B. Nash, M. P. Manfredi, B. Bozarth, and S. Howell, *Connecting with the New Healthcare Consumer: Defining Your Strategy* (New York: Aspen Publishers, 2001).

15. L. Harteker, "Partnerships for Patient Safety: Profiles of Four Hospitals," *Advances in Family-Centered Care* 9, no. 1 (2003): 17–26.

16. Council on Graduate Medical Education and National Advisory Council on Nurse Education and Practice, *Collaborative Education to Ensure Patient Safety* (Rockville, MD: Health Resources and Services Administration, 2000) [http://www.cogme.gov/jointmtg.htm]. Accessed October 2007.

17. A. Wrynn, "The History of American Health, Hygiene and Fitness," [http://personal.ecu.edu/estesst/2323/readings/americanpe.html]. Accessed December 2007.

18. S. R. Cruess, S. Johnston, and R. L. Cruess, "Professionalism for Medicine: Opportunities and Obligations," *Medical Journal of Australia* 177, no. 4 (2002): 208–11.

19. U.S. Department of Health and Human Services, *Informal Caregiving: Compassion in Action* (Washington, DC: HHS, 1998); National Family Caregivers Association, Random Sample Survey of Family Caregivers, Summer 2000, unpublished data.

20. F. R. Gaillour, "The 'Perfect Storm' in Healthcare: Crisis or Opportunity?" *HealthLeaders News*, January 6, 2003 [http://www.health leaders.com/news/feature1.php?contentid=40951]. Accessed July 2003.

21. National Patient Safety Foundation, "The Role of the Patient Advocate: A Consumer Fact Sheet" (2002) [http://www.npsf.org/pdf/paf/PatientAdvocate.pdf]. Accessed October 2007.

22. A. Richardson, "Infusion Pumps: The Views of Patients." Unpublished paper prepared for the National Patient Safety Agency (May 2003).

23. A. Hirschoff, ed., *The Family as Patient Care Partners: Leveraging Family Involvement to Improve Quality, Safety, and Satisfaction* (Washington, DC: Advisory Board Company, 2006).

24. Institute for Healthcare Improvement, "Health Care Leaders Leading: A Dana-Farber Cancer Institute Executive Describes the Crucial Role of Leadership in Driving Patient Safety" [http://www.ihi.org/IHI/Topics/PatientSafety/MedicationSystems/Improvement Stories/HealthCareLeadersLeadingADanaFarberCancerInstitute executivedescribesthecrucialroleofleadershipindriv.htm]. Accessed October 2007.

25. Children's Hospitals and Clinics of Minnesota, Family Advisory Council [http://www.childrensmn.org/Communities/FamilyAdvisory Council.asp]. Accessed October 2007.

26. M. Ringel, "Mistakes in Medicine," Nexus (March/April 2003) [http://www.nexuspub.com/articles/2003/march2003/zen_mar_2003.htm]. Accessed October 2007.

27. Council on Social Work Education, *Myths and Opportunities: An Examination of the Impact of Discipline—Specific Accreditation on Interprofessional Education* (Alexandria, VA: Council on Social Work Education, 1999), 3; Council on Graduate Medical Education and National Advisory Council on Nurse Education and Practice, *Collaborative Education to Ensure Patient Safety.*

28. E. H. O'Neil and the Pew Health Professions Commission, *Recreating Health Professional Practice for a New Century, the Fourth Report of the Pew Health Professions Commission* (San Francisco: Center for the Health Professions at the University of California, December 1998).

Infusion Pumps:
The Views of Patients*

Ann Richardson

Research Methodology

This research by the National Patient Safety Agency (NPSA) was limited to patients who had used an infusion pump during a stay in a hospital within the previous five years for pain or symptom control following an investigation, treatment, or surgery; chemotherapy; intravenous feeding; or insulin control because they were diabetics. All participants were recruited through organizations for people with cancer or diabetes, either via a mailing to members about the research or through local support group organizers. Some were found by word of mouth from other research participants.

A short description of the nature and purpose of the study was prepared for those to be interviewed. They were assured that the information would be treated as confidential and that their treatment would not be affected by a decision to take part. A topic guide was used, covering the experiences of patients from their initial use of an infusion pump to the point of completion. The interviews were tape recorded and transcribed verbatim. The information collected was carefully analyzed as a whole and by type of use. A copy of the research report was subsequently sent to all people interviewed for their comments.

*Unpublished paper prepared for the National Patient Safety Agency, United Kingdom, May 2003, and reprinted here by permission of the agency. Ann Richardson is patient experience and public involvement project manager, National Patient Safety Agency, London, England.

In all, 24 interviews were carried out, 13 in person and 11 by telephone. The participants were 7 men and 17 women, ranging in age from the early 20s to late 70s. In terms of diagnosis, 16 had cancer (or, in one case, a woman whose husband had died from cancer), 7 were people with diabetes (including 1 mother of a child with diabetes), and 1 had an unclear diagnosis. Of those with cancer, most had used a pump for more than one purpose: 13 for chemotherapy, 11 for morphine or other painkiller following an operation, and 3 for other purposes, such as intravenous feeding. The numbers involved in these respective categories were not purposively sought but simply emerged from the process of recruitment.

Study Results

Understanding the Infusion Pump

Almost all participants thought that it was important to understand as much as possible about their treatment, including the infusion pump. But there was considerable variation in the extent to which they were informed. Most of those having chemotherapy said that nurses tended to provide a lot of information while setting up the pump ("That's your time with them, when you have an opportunity to talk about it all"). Although much of this discussion centered on the drugs and their side effects, those who wanted information about the pump generally felt able to ask for it, with nurses ready to answer questions. On the other hand, a few would have liked to have had information earlier, because the first day of chemotherapy was "not a good day to ingest that information."

In contrast, those who used a pump for pain relief were often given little information or given it at the wrong time. A number said they could not remember being told anything about the pump but knew they must have been given some information because they understood the mechanics of controlling the dosage via the booster button. Some explicitly remembered a discussion about this. A few said they were given no information at all and felt quite shocked to wake up and find themselves attached to a pump. It was agreed that it could be difficult to find the right time for a discussion, as patients had other worries immediately before an operation and were too drowsy afterward.

The role of the booster button in the use of morphine was an issue on which clearer information was felt by patients to be particularly important. Two participants were hesitant to use their morphine fully for fear of addiction. One woman was very worried that the supply might run out and therefore tended to underdose herself ("I was very nervous of using up my quota and then not having pain relief for a long time afterward").

Participants were asked about the extent to which they had been informed about safety issues concerning the pump, such as the alarms, batteries, or need to avoid mobile phones; virtually no one could remember having been given any such details. Some said that they had seen notices about not using mobile phones because it could affect the equipment but were not clear about the details ("We were never told which equipment. I thought it was for people on ventilators").

Supervision of the Pump

Most participants believed that their pump was well supervised. Nurses were said to be "quite vigilant" and responded fairly quickly when alarms went off, especially for those on chemotherapy. But some people were less content with the speed of nursing attention, particularly those using a pump for pain control, where alarms were often not attended to quickly. Some said they had little sense that anyone was watching what was happening, and some had waited a long period for help. One woman, whose morphine had run out, said she was left for several hours in pain.

Because of the apparent difficulties of getting nurses' attention, a number of patients spoke of doing as much as they could for themselves, and one tried to help others. One woman indicated that she watched the nurses carefully and learned to adjust the pump for herself. Another spoke about the importance of mutual help by patients: "It's a terrifying scenario. The hospital relies on patients taking as much interest in each other as do the staff. You just pray to God that someone would help you if you ran into difficulties."

But some people thought it was potentially dangerous for patients to get involved in technical aspects of the pump.

Practical Problems

Patients tended to have strong views about the cannula. Many commented that it was very painful to insert and that nurses often did not get it right the first time. Some nurses were much more successful than others ("There were one or two that had the knack"); it was particularly worrisome to patients when nurses got flustered or panicky in an unsuccessful attempt. Patients varied in their willingness to refuse treatment from what they believed to be the less competent staff, whereas a number wished to and some did, and at least one did not refuse because she did not want to give offense.

A few people spoke of being pleasantly surprised when a cannula was inserted easily. In one case, for instance, a nurse used a very small needle with much reduced pain, and the patient then wondered why these were not used all the time ("Had they ordered all these particular sizes, and they had to be used?"). Another patient found that one nurse used a better location for the insertion, making it not at all painful.

Many participants disliked the physical restrictions imposed by a cannula. One man described lying in bed "like a statue" at first because of fear of pulling it out. Others talked about the difficulty of performing ordinary tasks, such as getting out of bed, eating, or reading, when one needed to move the hand and arm. The pulling of the needle entailed in such activity could be the source of some anxiety ("You feel that prick and you think maybe it's gone through the wall of the vein or something").

A number of patients found the pump's movable stand to be awkward to maneuver, especially over stepped areas or through doors, and they were conscious of needing to take great care not to trip over the wires ("It's a complete art form being able to walk around with one of those—any cancer survivor's a Fred Astaire by the end of it"). Some people commented that moving around involved a lot of palaver, sometimes because an alarm would go off accidentally and sometimes because of the sheer amount of equipment involved ("Everything came with you— you went up and down these stairs looking like something from Venus"). But most participants learned to move around over time and some never found moving to be a problem.

Emotional Needs and Support

Perhaps most strikingly, a number of patients spoke about their often neglected emotional needs associated with the pump. They stressed that finding themselves in need of such treatment was itself difficult, and the pump only served to underline the seriousness of their situation: "Faced with these pumps and things, emotionally it was a big shock. . . . I could see my life changing. You never think you're going to have to be wired up to one of these machines and have drugs pumped into you."

But the pump itself gave rise to considerable anxiety, often because of misunderstandings about how it worked. For instance, a common source of worry was seeing air bubbles in the tube, as people had understood from television programs that air bubbles in their bloodstream were dangerous ("The first time I saw an air bubble, I remember being totally petrified. I thought, 'Right, that is it—you are a goner!'"). A similar concern was seeing blood backed up into the pump, which several people found disquieting.

Moreover, some people intensely disliked the sense of being attached to a piece of equipment. It gave them a feeling of being "tethered" ("It's like being a prisoner with a ball and chain around your foot. . . . I felt quite claustrophobic at times"). One woman noted that this did not matter so much when she was ill but was irritating as she became better. One man found it disconcerting that the pump faced away from him, as he felt himself connected to an "alien" thing; this fear would have been eased if he could have seen it.

Perhaps the most worrying event was hearing the alarm attached to an infusion pump, especially the first time. This was not only very annoying ("It could go wrong eight times in a night—you'd be just going back to sleep and it would bleep again; sometimes I felt like throwing the machine out of the window"), but it could also be a source of real panic among those who assumed that it indicated a crisis. Moreover, the fact that the alarms went off frequently raised a fundamental issue of patient safety, because everyone began to ignore them: "The alarm is almost more redundant than a burglar alarm in a house with the neighbors ignoring it—imagine, if there had been a real problem here and we were just ignoring it."

The emotional responses of a few patients, it might be added, were more positive. Two said that they came to view the pump as a "friend" because it was providing important pain relief or treatment.

Safety

This study was commissioned with an interest in patient safety, and participants recounted a number of incidents, most of which arose from human error. Two patients had their lines severely pulled on or pulled out accidentally; one line got caught in a vacuum cleaner and another was pulled out by a nurse while the pump was being rigged up ("It was extraordinarily painful; I just had surgery that morning"). One woman's Hickman line was wrongly unscrewed one night so that it fell apart onto the floor the next morning. After 15 seconds during which the patient couldn't breathe, the nurse managed to screw it back again. The same woman also suffered a nurse's trying to flush an antibiotic into the line neat rather than diluted. Fortunately, her husband noted that something seemed wrong and stopped the procedure.

One woman believed that her diabetic daughter was put at risk because of ignorance about diabetes on the part of the nursing staff. Soon after setting up an insulin pump, the nurses asked her about the appropriate rate ("One nurse seemed to think that if the blood sugar was low, you needed more insulin; she had it totally the wrong way around—and that was scary"). A possible seizure was averted only because an endocrinologist happened to be on the ward and adjusted the pump appropriately.

A few experiences arose from nurses' apparently not concentrating on the matter at hand. One patient experienced an inaccurately inserted cannula and as a result was burned by chemotherapy drugs. Another had antisickness drugs put into the cannula in the wrong direction because a nurse was chatting with someone. Another patient found that her chemotherapy was not going through because the nurse had set the pump incorrectly. Two people had regular difficulties reaching their call button; one wife noted that nurses placed it out of reach every time they made her husband's bed.

One patient was highly concerned about a general lack of cleanliness, stating that nurses didn't wash their hands between patients and that the hospital itself was very unclean. It had been stressed to her that she should be kept very clean because of her neutropenia, yet the ward was quite dirty: "They give you advice about keeping clean, keeping away from animals, and instructing you to live in sterile conditions. And you're sitting in a ward watching cockroaches going across the floor, and you pick up dirt like you wouldn't believe. All the wards are splattered with blood, and the toilets weren't clean."

None of the patients had lodged a formal complaint about safety concerns presumably because of a reluctance to be a bother or to single out one nurse among an otherwise good team. There was also a concern about the possible consequences of rocking the boat: "When you've got to be there all the time, you don't want to fall out with any nurse or put any blame on anybody. Obviously, all the nurses stick together. And you hope it won't happen again."

Other Nursing Issues

A major concern for a number of participants was an apparent lack of knowledge among nurses about infusion pumps. The patients were disconcerted by the nurses' own hesitancies: "It was two [nurses] fumbling about that didn't seem to know what they were doing; they were saying, 'Do you think this is right?' and 'I'm not sure about this'—and you're thinking 'Oh, dear.'"

The handling of morphine was also an issue. One large man who found that the normal dose of morphine had limited effect after a major operation was distressed that nurses were unable to alter his dose, and he had to wait for a doctor. Three participants felt that they had become addicted to morphine. Although none blamed this on the nursing staff, they argued that the subsequent withdrawal of morphine was not handled well ("They just took it off and took it away and that was that"). Indeed, two suffered severe withdrawal symptoms, one on a regular basis because she was in and out of the hospital frequently ("I suffered cold turkey every time I came out of hospital without really knowing why").

A number of comments were offered about the general nursing care. Some patients couldn't praise nurses highly enough ("They were very, very caring—absolutely brilliant, cheerful, and positive"). But many participants noted that the nurses were overworked and stressed. Although some patients were sympathetic to the difficulties, others felt less so, especially when the nurses themselves were moody. One man aptly summarized the general problem: "The good nurses are run off their feet, whereas the others are standing around talking."

Coming Off the Pump

Coming off the pump was generally a fairly straightforward experience. Most people said that they knew what was happening, although there was little explanation ("They just came along and disconnected it"). Several spoke of the sense of release when they came off the pump ("It's the biggest relief you can imagine—you are free again"). Two people found it annoying that the cannula was not removed until just before they left the hospital, although they could see the reason for it. Few people felt there were problems associated with the removal of the cannula, but one man said removing the associated tape was painful.

Issues for Diabetic Regular Insulin Pump Users

The participants who were regular insulin pump users raised completely different issues. For them, the principal problem was not coming to terms with new equipment but rather getting the hospital staff to allow them to use their own pump while they were in the hospital. Four patients had managed to do so and were very appreciative of this decision ("It was very much a case of 'you know what to do with your pump, so if you're happy, we won't mess about in any way, unless there is an emergency'"). In most cases, the use of the patient's own pump had been preceded by some discussion between the patient and hospital staff, sometimes with considerable resistance from some staff.

These patients were concerned, however, about the ability of hospital staff to cope with their pumps (for instance, if they were under an anesthetic) because of a lack of familiarity with the pumps. Several patients brought detailed written information together with the phone number for a diabetes support team. But they did note an eagerness to learn ("I had everybody and their granny coming to look at it. . . . I had to tell them what I was doing and why I was doing it. They were all fascinated").

On five separate occasions, one participant had been required to use hospital equipment during her operation. She ascribed this to ignorance on the part of hospital staff, but she intensely disliked having decisions made for her ("It's not even a discussion between yourself and the doctors—it's 'you do what they say' and that's it").

Conclusions and Recommendations

Probably the most common recommendation among the research participants was for better training for nurses on how to work with and around infusion pumps. It was suggested that this should apply to all nurses, even those who would not normally handle a pump, so they could know how to cope in an emergency.

Some of this training should be on technical matters. Nurses should be trained to check that pumps are functioning properly so that they are not found to be faulty at the last minute. Nurses should also ensure that patients on pumps always have access to their call button (for instance, by looping the cord over the patient's hand). One woman, who had worked in television, spoke of a rule that no one ever stepped across a camera operator's cable and suggested there should be a similar rule about not stepping over any line connecting patients to equipment. The diabetic participants on regular insulin pumps argued that nursing staff needed to gain more familiarity with these pumps, possibly through more focused discussions with users.

More attention to the emotional needs of patients was thought to be equally important. Participants indicated that nurses should understand that being on a pump is an unusual experience, and patients may require considerable reassurance. Nurses also need to understand patients' fears concerning pumps and should be trained to appreciate a patient's sense of confinement. Two people suggested that nurses should be required to experience this for a day or two ("just to see what it's like").

Many participants stressed the need for fuller information about their disease and treatment. This information should also be imparted to the main caregiver whenever possible. It should include information about the pump—why patients were having one, how it operates, how long patients would be having it, the dosage, likely problems, and the details of its use. Participants also suggested that patients be given ample warning about issues likely to worry them, such as air bubbles and the alarms. A system for collecting and disseminating ideas from patients on how to cope with a pump would be helpful.

This early research by the NPSA serves as a good indicator of the benefit of listening to patients' views, as it raised new and important issues for consideration. The NPSA is currently developing information for patients and a training program for nurses on infusion pumps.

2

The Patient's Role in Safety: A Physician's Perspective

Joel Mattison, MD

The past half century has seen incredible changes in medicine as well as in the world at large. Recently, a "great awakening" seems to be entering medical ranks. Those of us in medicine are now more willing to learn from other disciplines and industries. There is less sensitivity about protecting our profession from public scrutiny and criticism. The very essence of medicine, the patient-doctor relationship, is undergoing considerable adjustment. Having practiced as a surgeon for many years, I have experienced all aspects of this transformation, and, like many physicians, I initially yearned for the good old days. Like anyone dealing with change, my understanding and acceptance of the revolution in medical practice was not a discrete, single event. I gradually moved from being uninterested (precontemplation stage) to considering the changes (contemplation stage) to deciding and preparing to adjust (action stage). These stages must be understood and heeded if we are to avoid becoming dinosaurs.

For the most part, the dominance of the medical model effectively suppressed the voice of the health care consumer. Paternalism was probably one of the most significant and yet subtle influences standing in the way of doctor-patient communication. And yet, like many in my profession, I saw no compelling need to relinquish the paternalistic role. In the early 1990s, I wrote a review of a motion picture, *The Doctor*, for the *Journal of the American Medical Association*. This film was an adaptation of the book *A Taste of My Own Medicine*, by

Dr. Edward E. Rosenbaum, originally published by Random House in 1988. In the book, Rosenbaum, a rheumatologist in Portland, Oregon, recounted his experiences undergoing treatment for cancer of the larynx. He wrote about his frustrations with the medical system, which included a delay in his diagnosis and a frequent display of indifference and lack of compassion by physicians and other caregivers. At the end of the 1991 movie version of this book, the physician (played by William Hurt) is both recovered and converted and in the last scene is requiring his residents to spend 72 hours as hospital patients as part of their medical training.

Needless to say, my review of Rosenbaum's book moved me further along toward the action stage in my professional transformation. It was hard not to appreciate the significance of the patient's point of view as recounted by Rosenbaum. At about this same time, the Picker/Commonwealth Program for Patient-Centered Care was established at Boston's Beth Israel Hospital and the Harvard Medical School. Initial research by this group culminated in the publication of the groundbreaking book by Margaret Gerteis, Susan Edgman-Levitan, Jennifer Daley, and Thomas L. Delbanco, *Through the Patient's Eyes* (San Francisco: Jossey-Bass, 1993). Not long after its publication, the *Journal of the American Medical Association* regularly began to publish patients' stories in the "A Piece of My Mind" column, and similar patient testimonials were published in other medical journals. The era of patient-centered care was in full swing, and many physicians, including myself, were becoming convinced that the voice of the patient deserved greater attention. Studies of consumer attitudes supported this sentiment. In one such study, physician-patient communication was identified by 57 percent of American respondents as an essential indicator of quality.[1]

But does the patient have a role to play in reducing medical errors? There is proven value to involving patients in medical decision making, yet the merit of patient involvement in the safety movement may still be an enigma for many physicians. I doubt if a patient would be able to prevent an inadvertent intraoperative injury or notice that the surgical sponge count was inaccurate. Even in cases of a delayed diagnosis, it would be unlikely that a layperson could immediately recognize and correct the clinician's error.

When the issue of patient safety comes up, physicians commonly envision incidents attributable to inappropriate practitioner decisions or actions. I agree that the average patient wouldn't have sufficient knowledge or the ability to prevent such mistakes from being made. On the other hand, the medical profession has heard repeatedly over the past several years that errors most often result from a complex interplay of multiple factors and only rarely are due to the carelessness, perversity, or misconduct of single individuals. The patient is one of the players in this complex system of care, and yet we often think of patients in a passive way as the victims of errors and safety failures.

Patients can play an active part in preventing mistakes and ensuring their own safety if given the correct information and the right tools for the job. For example, when the doctor discusses common medication side effects with a patient, the patient is better prepared to recognize unexpected problems.

Described in the remainder of this chapter are approaches that physicians and other health care providers can use to involve patients actively in error prevention. Some of these suggestions originate from my professional experiences as a surgeon and my administrative work in clinical resource management at St. Joseph's Hospital of St. Joseph's–Baptist Health Care in Tampa, Florida. In addition, not long ago I had the opportunity to view the health care system as a patient. This perspective made me realize the importance of strengthening the medical profession's resolve to collaborate with patients. It wasn't until I became a surgical patient that I fully realized the significance of the phrase "nothing about me, without me," a phrase reported to be first voiced by an English midwife at a Salzburg seminar in 1988.[2]

Involving Patients in Safety

Patient participation in health care safety improvement must start with dialogue. The word *dialogue* comes from the Greek word *dialogos*. *Dia* means "through," and *logos* means "the word" or "the principle behind the spoken word." Dialogue is different from discussion. When two people or groups are dialoguing, the goal is collaboration, with everyone involved coming out winners. In a discussion, each person or group is trying to convince the other of the correctness of an opinion or a position. Simply put, effective dialogue can allow clinicians and patients to put aside the traditional dominance-subordination structure to achieve the common goal of safety.

It is important to use creative thinking and approaches that facilitate real two-way communication between providers and patients. Although certainly worthwhile, simply putting a patient or two on a health service advisory committee is clearly not sufficient to ensure meaningful dialogue. To improve the safety of health care services, we need to involve as many voices as possible, the pleasant (those who agree with us) and the not so pleasant (those who don't). Only by sharing all possible solutions to the safety problems in health care will substantial improvements be made. Physicians and other professionals must help patients understand what is needed from them in order to make the health care experience safer. Next, providers must find out what patients need to feel safe.

Helping Patients Understand Their Role

The long and often challenging process of sharing information and making it meaningful for patients has several aspects. Like many hospitals, St. Joseph's in Tampa distributes patient brochures to facilitate communication. Everyone entering as an inpatient is given the Patient Information Guide before leaving the admitting office. Included in the guide is a page entitled "10 Tips to Help Us Keep You Safe" (see figure 2-1).

Figure 2-1.   Safety Suggestions in the Patient Information Guide at St. Joseph's Hospital, Tampa, Florida

10 Tips to Help Us Keep You Safe:

Research has shown that the best way to prevent medical errors is for patients and families to take an active part in their medical care. You can play an important role by following these simple tips.

1. Make sure every health care team member who cares for you checks your name band. Please help us by keeping your identification bracelet in place until discharge.

2. Ask us any questions you may have. Discuss your concerns. Ask a family member or friend to speak for you if you are not able to speak for yourself.

3. Let us help you out of bed until we know you are steady on your feet. We do not want you to fall.

4. Give us complete and correct information about your health history, personal habits (such as alcohol use or smoking), and diet.

5. Make sure we know what medicine(s) you take. This includes what is ordered by a doctor and what you take on your own (such as aspirin or cold remedies). Include vitamins, herbs, and diet supplements.

6. Ask what each medicine is for. Learn about medicine side effects. Tell us if you think you are having a side effect.

7. Find out why a test or treatment is needed and how it may help you.

8. Ask your doctor about the results of your tests. Do not assume that "No news is good news."

9. Feel free to ask health care team members if they have washed their hands before they provide care to you. Good hand washing is still the best simple way to prevent the spread of germs.

10. Be sure you know what to expect when you go home and know what to report to your doctor.

Source: Publications Department, St. Joseph's Hospital, Tampa, Florida. Reprinted with permission.

In addition to these ten tips, I would like to add some particular, individualized examples of one-on-one suggestions that caregivers could offer hospitalized patients.

1. Make yourself easily and instantly recognizable and not just the patient in "B bed." Using a black wide-tip felt marker, print your name in large letters on a thick (card stock) sheet of white paper that is at least $8\frac{1}{2} \times 11$ inches. Do not use longhand or ornamental styles in writing your name. Do not add other information to the sign, even if you think it would be helpful to your caregivers. Tape or otherwise affix this sign to the head of your hospital bed or to the wall above the head of the bed. This sign provides one more way for caregivers to identify you.

2. If an anesthesiologist visits you prior to a surgery, tell him or her about any medications that you have been taking, even if you have stopped taking them. This is particularly important for medications containing steroids. Some effects of steroids continue for months after being discontinued. It is necessary for the anesthesiologist and any other treating physicians to know any history of steroid usage to avoid potential serious problems.

3. Some patients mistakenly assume that food allergies won't be a problem during the hospital stay. Although this seems to bear witness to a patient's trust in the system, it is important that the hospital caregivers are told about any food allergies. It is easier to avoid the problem than to treat it after it becomes full blown.

4. Everyone tends to forget things, and the stress of being a patient in the hospital may make the tendency even worse. Keep a small notepad and pencil at your bedside to jot down thoughts that might otherwise be lost during those temporary memory lapses.

Physicians must also share with patients the often difficult and sensitive issue of the potential for individual mistakes (for example, wrong-site surgery, diagnosis delays, incorrect medication prescriptions). We must help our patients to understand these potentials so that they may help us to guard against them.

What can a patient do to decrease the likelihood that practitioners will make a mistake? From the standpoint of reducing wrong-site surgeries, it is frequently valuable to give the patient a brochure describing the procedure (or even a general brochure on all procedures). In addition, proper informed consents and written operative permits can be effective safeguards if patients are encouraged to speak up with questions or concerns.

Reducing unnecessary risk exposure through the use of multiple safeguards can eliminate many errors, yet it is not always an easy thing to do. Ideally, each process has repeated checks to ensure that everything is proceeding correctly. For example, a nurse comes to the patient's hospital bedside with a pink pill. The patient asks, "Is this my heart medicine?" The nurse's answer is, "Yes." Patient: "How do you know?" Nurse: "I got it out of a labeled stock bottle." Patient persists, "How do you know that the bottle was labeled correctly and the drug was not past the expiration date?" And so on. We eventually come to some point in the process at which further checks would be absurd or at least not helpful (e.g., "How do you know that the source of this digoxin is real foxglove?"). At such a point, we have to accept the source or else trust that the information we have is correct or at least adequate.

A similar interaction can transpire when the patient asks the clinician, "How do you know who I am?" or "How do I know who you are?" or "How do you know what is in the pill cup?" There is some point at which one has to settle for the best available information and depend on common sense. Knowing one from the other is a matter of judgment. Tina Long, a nurse known for her excellence at St. Joseph's Hospital, once put it this way: "I think that we eventually just have to stop at some reasonable point and say, 'I believe that we have enough information to go ahead and give this medication.'" The human race is so interdependent that in some instances we can only move forward on the basis of well-founded trust.

When we think about inpatient safety, the subject of delirium (acute confusional state) in elderly hospitalized patients comes up only rarely. Delirium, however, is common and a serious source of morbidity and mortality among older hospitalized patients. If we are interested in safety, we can ill afford to ignore the following facts. Delirium can be caused or aggravated by cognitive impairment, sleep deprivation, immobility, visual impairment, hearing impairment, and dehydration.[3] Primary prevention is probably the most effective treatment strategy. Despite our best efforts, however, confusion will still continue to be a problem for some patients. In these situations, the patient's family or friends should be actively recruited to serve as safety advocates on the patient's behalf. But even young, relatively healthy patients may be unable to fully participate in error prevention activities. That may be why nearly half of the consumer participants in a recent unpublished study at St. Joseph's Hospital said that it is best to have family or friends on hand to monitor care.

Seeking and Using Patient Feedback

It is not uncommon to find in the "Patient Rights and Responsibilities" statement given to hospitalized patients a sentence like, "We will provide the best health care possible in a safe, clean, quiet, and pleasant environment." This promise is found under the heading of facility responsibilities, but there is usually no corollary statement listed in the patient rights section. Shouldn't we be telling patients that they have the right to feel safe while receiving care at the hospital? Perhaps that is what we think we are saying when we ask patients to answer questions completely so that clinicians can provide better care.

We probably cannot tell patients too often that health care team members use the identification bracelet on their wrist to confirm patient identity before medications are given or treatments initiated. Does cautioning patients to always call the nurse for help in getting out of bed help them feel safe? I would think so, but I can't say for sure. This brings us to the second component of effective dialogue: seeking feedback from patients and using it to create a safer environment.

Physicians and other health care professionals must avoid stereotyped thinking about what makes patients feel safe. When the dialogue is only one sided, all we have is a discussion in which medical professionals try to convince patients to give us what we need to keep them safe. To turn this discussion into a dialogue, we have to discover from patients what they need from us to feel safe. Patients and medical professionals don't always have the same ideas about the relative importance of safety issues. These differences became apparent when St. Joseph's–Baptist Health Care started asking patients about their safety concerns.[4] The feedback commonly falls into the following six general categories:

1. *Universal precautions:* Caregivers not washing hands, not wearing personal protective equipment, not following isolation protocols, etc.
2. *Sharps:* Sharps containers overflowing, needles left in room from a previous patient, needle cap found in bed, etc.
3. *Medications:* Nurses not washing hands, not checking patient's identification band prior to medication administration, not explaining the purpose for medications, etc.
4. *Shower/bath:* Not clean, too much clutter, dirty bedside commode, etc.
5. *Cleanliness:* Dirty bathroom, dirty patient room, dirty privacy curtains, etc.
6. *Slip/trip/fall/clutter:* Too much clutter in halls and bathroom, uneven gravel on outdoor paths, uneven floor surfaces at door entryways, etc.

Many of these safety concerns are not the dramatic ones that most medical professionals would view as a high priority, yet this is what patients notice and tell us about in our questionnaire. Patients seem more focused on safety issues than on error issues (such as wrong-site surgery). This, of course, could be a very subtle and interesting form of denial. However, the survey results do heighten our awareness of what makes patients feel safe. Issues that draw the most attention from patients fall into the slip/trip/fall/clutter category. A preliminary goal for our hospital is to learn which categories of safety concerns receive the greatest number of comments from patients and then to resolve these concerns. In addition, the feedback has made us realize that patients need help in understanding the error aspects of safety that are worthy of their attention. The patient safety movement will not be complete if the patient perspective is not brought into the dialogue. The patient must be involved in many aspects of health care service that have an impact on safety, such as the following:

- Helping to reach an accurate diagnosis
- Deciding on an appropriate treatment or management strategy
- Choosing a suitably experienced and safe provider (with current appropriate certification and verified training)
- Ensuring that treatment is appropriately administered, monitored, and adhered to
- Identifying side effects or adverse events quickly and taking appropriate action[5]

By dialoguing with patients, the flow of information can go in both directions. Ultimately, this will have a positive impact on both safety and error-related concerns.

Improving Safety from the Ground Up

In any project, the greatest judgment is required in deciding how far back toward zero to take any existing system for which improvement is intended. This is true for the restoration of antiques and classic cars, for almost any complex surgical case, and for any finely tuned business enterprise. How far back does one go in removing old paint, what is to be done with rusted or dented hardware, and how does one decide when or whether to replace or repair? If, in restoration, one removes too much of the real thing, it may be analogous to the collector who was perhaps overly proud of owning George Washington's original axe, adding that it had had two heads and five handles but was still completely original.

The February 2003 issue of *Trustee* magazine carried an article about the $55 million replacement facility being built by St. Joseph's Community Hospital in West Bend, Wisconsin.[6] The new hospital building, which was completed in May 2005, was designed for improved patient safety. "Spaces clearly have an impact on safety," said St. Joseph's Community Hospital Chief Executive Officer John Reiling. "We looked at the relationship between technology, equipment, and the physical plant and their impact on each other. How could we translate this information to design around patient safety?"

To answer this question, a "learning lab" was sponsored with the University of Minnesota's Carlson School of Management. In attendance were more than two dozen patient safety experts; local and national leaders in health care administration, research, and systems engineering; human behavior researchers; hospital quality improvement professionals; accreditation specialists; medical educators; hospital architects; nurses; pharmacists; and physicians. Hospital planners have traditionally decided on the physical layout first when designing a new building, but in the learning lab, participants were taught how to look at processes before deciding on space—playing out how technology and structure could best assist those processes. In designing the new building, St. Joseph's Hospital in West Bend started with a list of the following top ten priorities:

1. Failure analysis should be ongoing.
2. Stakeholder input is critical.

3. Accountable leadership is needed to drive the process.

4. Design should focus on organizational processes.

5. Design should reflect an understanding of human factors.

6. Design should occur with vulnerable populations in mind.

7. Design should be flexible enough to accommodate change.

8. Design should be standardized whenever possible.

9. Design should facilitate immediate access to information.

10. Design should address known threats to patient safety.

Unfortunately, few health care organizations are given the opportunity to start from scratch. It is often hard just to take the dramatic step of discarding some of the oldest of the old and embracing the affordable new. It is clear, however, that this new kind of thinking and planning is the wave of the future. For the present, many organizations will have to compromise somewhat and look for patient safety improvements wherever they can be achieved, even in small increments.

Engendering a Passion for Safety

Safety awareness is not communicated by rote or rules alone. Inspiration and example are a start, but these are only successful when safe habits have permeated our beings, etched our souls, and become second nature. For example, those of us in surgery cannot force ourselves to scratch our noses after we have scrubbed and gowned up. This is an unforgivable sin, and compliance was ingrained while our paint was still wet. We are also unable to cross that thin red line in an operating suite in street clothes. This is such a fervent conviction that it never comes to mind to question why. Whether something bad will happen is moot, because crossing the line is simply unthinkable.

Seeing clinicians compulsively stop to wash their hands before entering a patient's room spreads the idea that this safe practice is woven into our lives and that everyone is working to keep the environment clean. Changes in behavior and attitude come about not through signs or repetition alone but through teaching by example. Someone once asked Albert Schweitzer if example was the best way of teaching, to which he replied, "It is the only way." His hospital at Lambaréné, in western Gabon, was built on this principle, and his patients largely followed his example (and that of his staff). Many arguments on nearly all subjects at Lambaréné were settled with the reminder in Schweitzer's own words, "It is commanded that we not do that."[7] Hardly a day would pass without someone repeating this to a patient, employee, or visitor, and I cannot recall anyone ever disputing this simple statement.

Is your hospital "littered"? What patients see as litter may (to us) mean only some variant of untidiness, whereas to patients every damp spot represents a urine spill and is a symbol of carelessness and an ominous warning sign. The only way to combat littered hallways is by precept and example. Health care professionals must create the impression that it is a sacrilege either to drop trash or to pass it by when it is in one's path. Patients and staff who see senior staff stop to pick up trash get the idea that everyone is working to keep the environment clean and safe.

A special word about "wet litter," or spills, leaks, and puddles: In addition to contributing to the appearance of slovenliness, these are a constant source of falls for patients and staff alike. Another, very small action can transform a patient's experience: covering the patient, especially during transit. However uncomfortable may be shivering in a cold hall and however embarrassing is the humiliation of being exposed, from the patient's viewpoint it is probably the indignity of being uncovered in a hallway that is most disturbing. Of course, it is important to prevent injury to patients, but attention to their dignity is a means of communicating concern. Caring for the whole patient is an element of safety often under-rated by medical professionals but highly valued by patients. Did you ever notice how litter-borne edentulous patients always draw the sheet up to cover their toothless mouths? These are only a few examples of the ways in which health care professionals can help patients to understand that we are a caring family in a safe facility. In many organizations, these behaviors and attitudes require a cultural change. Schweitzer's constant references to "reverence for life" were always evidence of his caring and respect for all living things.

Elaine Fantle Shimberg of Tampa, Florida, has written some sixteen helpful books for patients. She usually works with a medical expert, and her information is understandable, well organized, and trustworthy. One of her best books, co-authored with Dr. Sheldon Blau, is *How to Get Out of the Hospital Alive* (New York: Macmillian, 1997). This is not necessarily a book you'd want to give to an anxious friend who is just now entering the hospital for surgery. But it is certainly a book that will be an indispensable complement to your medical knowledge as you learn how patients think and react at a very vulnerable time. Read it with an open mind; it is filled with truths that physicians altogether too often think are beneath their notice.

Encouraging Provider-Patient Dialogue

Leading patients to see the importance of their attention to, and understanding of, their contribution to safety is a relatively new challenge for the medical profession. We must learn what seems most important to patients if we seriously covet their cooperation in eliminating or minimizing the potential for error. The principles of teaching by example are probably always the best solution to this problem. The medical professional must genuinely solicit patients' opinions and seek patients' informed cooperation. As we come to learn, understand, and accept more of the theories of error, and as we learn how to share this information with our patients, we can look forward to safer days and safer environments for all of us. All health care professionals must remain open and inquisitive about the viewpoints of those for whom it is our special privilege to care in a time of need.

Consumer involvement in the patient safety movement is an imperative. The public and our patients need to understand the risk in health services and participate with us in reducing that risk. At times this means forming partnerships with other physicians or nurses, for example, in improving medication safety and avoiding wrong-site surgery. At other times it means becoming educated consumers and realizing that there may be trade-offs between patient comfort and increased risk, as in the case of conscious sedation.

Patient safety will not be improved until everyone acknowledges that risks exist at all levels of health care. A safer way of caring for patients can be achieved by detecting, measuring, and monitoring risk, accompanied by steadfast determination. Safety is a continually evolving property of a complex system, especially a system as complex as modern medical care. It is a certainty that the sources of harm will change as medical care changes. Safety will be a never-ending, but important, aspect of the medical professional's work. The good news is that it can be one of those true "win-win-win" situations for our patients, for all of us who deliver health care, and for our provider institutions.

What a lot of sick compulsivity and extra effort we're talking about here! Keep in mind, however, that safety is the end result of unbridled altruism and never-fading enthusiasm. But if that is not reason enough, remember that you are a part of designing medical safety policy that may someday be a matter of life or death to you or your family. As a card-carrying member of society, remember that the life you save by some degree of excessive compulsivity may be your own. Is this too much trouble? I doubt it. The elevator is here and waiting at the bottom floor. Join in, and let's go up together.

References

1. Kaiser Family Foundation and Agency for Healthcare Research and Quality, *National Survey on Americans as Health Care Consumers: An Update on the Role of Quality Information* (Menlo Park, CA: Henry J. Kaiser Family Foundation, 2000).

2. National Patient Safety Foundation, *National Agenda for Action: Patients and Families in Patient Safety* (Chicago: National Patient Safety Foundation, 2003).

3. S. K. Inouye, S. T. Bogardus, Jr., P. A. Charpentier, L. Leo-Summers, D. Acampora, T. R. Holford, and L. M. Cooney, Jr., "A Multicomponent Intervention to Prevent Delirium in Hospitalized Older Patients," *New England Journal of Medicine* 340, no. 9 (1999): 669–76.

4. The St. Joseph's–Baptist system (St. Joseph's Emergency Center, South Florida Baptist Hospital, St. Joseph's Hospital, St. Joseph's Children's Hospital, and St. Joseph's Women's Hospital) has a total of 910 inpatient beds.

5. C. A. Vincent and A. Coulter, "Patient Safety: What about the Patient?" *Quality and Safety in Health Care* 11 (2002): 76–80.

6. L. Larson, "Putting Safety in the Blueprint," *Trustee* 56, no. 2 (2003): 9–13.

7. J. Mattison, "Lessons from Lambarene, Part I," *Bulletin of the American College of Surgeons* 77, no. 9 (1999): 10–21.

3

Creating Opportunities
for Patient Involvement

Paula S. Swain and Patrice L. Spath

A father is observed racing down a hospital hallway while talking on a cell phone. His anxiety is obvious as he advises the listener, "Do not let them give the baby anything until you see the vial that the medicine comes in."

This is an example of the consumer's fear response to media reports of unsafe health care situations. Alerts abound advising consumers of how to conduct themselves if they want to live to tell about their health care experience. The worst-case scenarios seem to surface to the top, with the public hearing about the dangers of hospital-acquired infections, medication mix-ups, significant physical injuries, and unfortunate equipment failures. On any given day we read news stories of errors in blood and donor typing, surgical removal of the wrong body parts, instruments and sponges left behind following operative procedures, and every other type of medication error imaginable. Besides the tales of misadventure in the news media, a number of publicly available books describe the inner workings of health care. In one such book, *Complications,* physician-author Atul Gawande notes that whereas the public may think medicine is an orderly field of knowledge and procedure, it definitely is not. Gawande describes medicine as an imperfect science with constantly changing knowledge, uncertain information, and fallible individuals.[1]

Contrary to what the public may think, safety has always been a priority in health care. A number of safeguards, precautions, and process improvements are making health care delivery safer every day. Remarkably, only in the past few years has the patient safety movement encouraged the active involvement of patients. Patients were often viewed as the victims of errors and safety failures, but there is growing evidence that they have a role in promoting safety. When patients ask questions about their medications or an anticipated procedure, they are serving as safeguards in the system—a reminder to caregivers to recheck or validate that the right thing is being done.

Adding the patient to the health care system of checks and balances can help prevent what may have been a simple mistake from becoming a harmful error that reaches the patient. To gain the value of this additional safeguard, health care professionals must encourage patients to pay attention to the care being provided to them and speak up if something doesn't seem right. The act of clarification can serve as a "pause" in what might otherwise be a very complex or tightly coupled, high-risk process. A *tightly coupled process* is one in which the steps follow one another so closely that an error in one step cannot be recognized and responded to before the next step is well under way.[2]

Patients who know what to expect from the health care experience can check on the appropriate performance of clinical tasks. For example, practitioners should discuss the common side effects of a medication when prescribing something new for a patient. If such a discussion fails to occur, patients are ill prepared to cope with side effects and may not recognize unexpected problems. Failure to receive information about the side effects of a medication should prompt the patient to ask questions of the physician or pharmacist.

The health care industry has endorsed an active role for consumers in helping to reduce errors by encouraging patients to ask questions and be vigilant. In 2000, the American Hospital Association issued a Quality Advisory to its members urging them to improve medication safety by partnering with patients.[3] In 2002, the Joint Commission, together with the Centers for Medicare and Medicaid Services, launched a national program to encourage patients to take a role in preventing health care errors by becoming active, involved, and informed participants on the health care team.[4] In 2003, the National Patient Safety Foundation partnered with groups like the American Hospital Association and the American Medical Association to create brochures and fact sheets to educate consumers on such topics as "Preventing Infections in the Hospital—What You as a Patient Can Do."[5] In the same year, the Agency for Healthcare Research and Quality and the National Council on Patient Information and Education jointly released a new resource called "Your Medicine: Play It Safe" to help consumers use prescription medicines safely.[6]

While the number and variety of consumer involvement initiatives have increased significantly in the past few years, many patients are still reticent to act as safety partners with caregivers. A 2006 study of hospitalized patients found that very few helped mark their surgical incision site or asked about caregivers' hand-washing practices.[7] Despite being asked to participate in adverse event prevention, patients may have no doubts about their safety or disregard their doubts because they trust health care professionals to keep them safe.[8,9]

To more effectively engage patients as active partners in the patient safety movement, health care professionals must first understand how things look from the patient's perspective. Patients want to be treated like responsible adults capable of assimilating information, asking informed questions, and having reasonable expectations. Yet the health care experience often falls short of these expectations. Consider how one patient described her stay at a large urban hospital for treatment of sepsis.

It was late, about 11:45 PM, on the first night of my hospital admission. I'd been in the hospital for fourteen hours. My last recorded temperature was 103.2°F, and the first dose of antibiotic was just hung. The air in the room was still. The air-conditioning must have been off on this end of the hall. My husband was dozing in a chair by the bed. It is so hot that I can't breathe. My head is pounding and every inch of my body hurts.

I'm sure I will be left on my own tonight. At change of shift, the night nurse walked in and I requested "something" for my temperature and aching body, and air-conditioning. No one got back to me, so after an hour of waiting I used the call bell. "They" could not understand my request over the intercom and promised to come to my room. When the nurse stopped by and heard my request, she answered that she was pretty sure I had nothing ordered but would check. I suggested she call the physician for an order before it got too much later. Her body language told me I was on my own. I never saw her again.

I woke my husband and instructed him to get two rubber gloves from the box of rubber gloves in my room and go down to the nutrition room and fill each glove with ice. He was worried someone would confront him—I assured him no one would bother him at this late hour. Soon he came back with the gloves filled with ice. He quickly got the gist of cooling me and supplied me with towels to catch the melting ice dripping from my body. He found a basin and went back to the nutrition room and stocked up on more icy gloves.

Clearly, I "knew" too much, asked too many questions, was not the priority or whatever else was in the equation. I truly felt retaliated against and vowed I would do what I could on my own so I would not be sabotaged in my pursuit of health.

The patient, a registered nurse with previous bedside experience at another hospital, was forced by her illness to make the transition from caring for patients to being a patient herself. She found the stark realities of health care terrifying when viewed from the patient's vantage point. Her health care background would qualify her as an "activated patient"—a concept that emerged from work that has been done around the role of the patient in the so-called chronic disease model.[10] Activated patients are considered sufficiently informed and motivated to handle the day-to-day management of their chronic condition. Similar characteristics—informed and motivated—will help patients to be more effective partners in the patient safety movement. Yet as the patient's story of her hospitalization unfolds in this chapter, it will become apparent that the attitudes and actions of health care professionals must change if the goal of patient- and family-centered patient safety is to be realized.

New Attitudes and Actions

Health care providers now have access to a large array of patient safety materials that can be shared with patients. However, these materials will not meet the intended goal of consumer involvement in patient safety until practitioners and the health care system embrace patients as valuable and active partners. First and foremost, health care professionals must truly believe that patients have an important role in reducing mistakes in the delivery of health care services. The need to include patients in the process of care was one of the safety improvement principles advanced in the Institute of Medicine's 1999 report *To Err Is Human: Building a Safer Health System*.[11] In support of this principle, numerous medical professional groups, such as the American College of Physicians, have issued position statements describing the importance of involving patients in discussions and in the decision process.[12] The National Patient Safety Foundation is urging all hospitals, health systems, and national and local health care organizations to collaborate with patients and families in systems and patient safety programs.[13] Health care facilities accredited by the Joint Commission are expected to encourage patients/clients/residents to ask questions and express concerns about their own safety and to provide the means for doing so.[14]

The success of efforts to partner with patients and families for the purpose of improving safety will actually depend largely on the attitudes and actions of individual caregivers—not on health care consumers. It is fairly easy to embrace the concept of open and honest communication with patients to gain the information needed for diagnosis or treatment purposes. But what if those same patients question why the caregiver touched them without washing his or her hands first? Or question the need for a particular procedure? Will health care professionals be as accepting of collaboration when patients are challenging clinical practices or professional decisions? No one likes to have his or her judgment questioned, and the usual emotional response is to become defensive and angry. Consider how caregivers responded to questions asked by the patient hospitalized for treatment of sepsis.

I was told that I needed an infusion of a potent antibiotic to stop the sepsis that was forming in my body. However, because my peripheral veins were inadequate, I would need to have a percutaneous intravenous catheter (PIC line) inserted. The health care provider who installed the PIC line told me who should draw blood out of the catheter as well as how to manage the catheter before and after every antibiotic infusion. He also told me that this was the only access available to infuse the antibiotic, short of a more invasive procedure.

I felt responsible for assisting in maintaining the PIC line over the course of my treatment, which would take two weeks. I asked each new nurse that arrived to administer a dose of antibiotics if she or he had experience managing a PIC line. Another time I questioned a radiology technician who was planning to infuse contrast through the PIC line for a CT scan that had been ordered. When I asked questions, merely in an attempt to protect the PIC line, much of the time I was met with hostility and frustration by caregivers who reported that they were "just trying to do their jobs."

I got inconsistent messages from my caregivers and was worried about protecting the catheter. Thankfully, a thoughtful charge nurse finally put written instructions on how to maintain the PIC line on the door to my hospital room. This was after I'd taught fourteen different nurses how to manage that line. I don't know if the radiology technician learned anything from our exchange, but I ended up having a CT scan without any contrast agent.

Professional attitudes influence actions. Most patients are keen to take responsibility for playing their part in trying to optimize treatment outcomes; however, many are frustrated by the lack of caregiver support in allowing them to satisfactorily fulfill this role.[15] Health care professionals may feel confronted and become defensive when the patient asks a question. In this situation, patients can easily become concerned about the safety of the care they are receiving. Physicians, nurses, and other health care professionals must learn how to interact and support patients who question their care. An ancient Buddhist story illustrates the type of communication gap that may exist between patients and health care professionals:

> The King said: "Venerable Nagasena, will you converse with me?" Nagasena: "If your majesty will speak with me as wise men converse, I will; but if your majesty converses with me as kings converse, I will not." "How then converse with the wise, venerable Nagasena?" "The wise do not get angry when they are driven into a corner; kings do."[16]

In a patient-safe culture, health care professionals must converse like wise men, not kings, when responding to inquisitive patients and/or family members. Caregivers may need coaching as well as education to narrow the communication gap. No patient should be afraid to ask a question, and no practitioner should appear offended by a patient who is willing to speak up. It helps to understand that patients may set high expectations or ask frequent questions in response to their own feelings of being out of control. It is the health care professional's job to facilitate a process whereby patients can regain control by validating patients' concerns, providing reassurance, and finding legitimate ways for patients to be actively involved. Caregivers must also be clear on the expectation that patients should inquire whenever they believe that care is not being provided in a safe manner. Consider how staff responses to the septic patient varied immediately after admission to the hospital.

My physician had urged me to hurry in getting to the hospital so that treatment would get started right away for the infection in my leg. Transportation from admissions to my hospital room seemed efficient enough. Yet once I got to my room, I was left alone. It soon became apparent there were other issues being dealt with on the floor that were more important than the "new admission in 624"!

During the first three hours, a few of the various staff members looked into my room. I couldn't get even an aspirin out of the group. No physician orders had come in, and the staff members appeared willing to wait until orders were called in. I wondered why no one had the initiative to call my physician? The obvious conclusion: "The staff don't care." Shift change added to the confusion. I asked for the nurse caring for me, but no one would commit. Finally, I asked to fill out my own assessment form and start the plan of care. After that, a nurse described as an "admitting nurse" sat down to take my health history. We bonded. Even though she knew nothing of my physician's orders, she listened to me, observed my wound, and heard my anxiety.

Effective Communication

One way to better understand how to communicate with patients would be to revitalize bedside teaching in medical schools. For a number of reasons, actual teaching at the bedside has declined from an incidence of 75 percent in the 1960s to an incidence of less than 16 percent in 1997.[17] Bedside teaching in medical schools, as in other settings of learning, is very well suited for using role modeling as a technique for teaching patient collaboration strategies. Although it is possible to describe appropriate communication skills, it is far more effective to demonstrate those skills through interactions with actual patients. Adults attach more meaning to learning gained from actual experience than that gained from passive learning.[18] And several studies have shown that a majority of patients enjoy the bedside teaching experience and feel that it helps them better understand their conditions.[19]

Some of the principles and benefits of the bedside teaching experience are evident in the collaborative practice models of patient care that hospitals and other health care providers are implementing. For example, "interdisciplinary rounding" is a component of the collaborative care model in the cardiac surgery unit at Concord Hospital in Concord, New Hampshire.[20] Members of the cardiac care team come together at one time each day to make rounds at each patient's bedside. Family members are encouraged to be present, and the patient and family members are encouraged to participate in the rounds process. Every effort is made to speak in ordinary language instead of medical terminology. In addition to discussing the patient's progress and treatment plan, the patient, family members, and cardiac care team members are asked about anything that didn't go as expected, or "system glitches." Ever since the morning rounds process was implemented, patients and family members have reported knowing exactly what is happening and what is planned. At first, practitioners felt uncomfortable discussing clinical situations openly with patients and family members and accepting their input. With time, however, participants became more at ease, and now practitioners frequently comment about how rewarding the rounds process is and how much it means to patients and families.

Health care professional groups are developing hands-on training resources to teach their members the communication skills that are important in creating an understanding and trusting relationship with patients. The American Academy of Orthopaedic Surgeons (AAOS) was one of the first medical associations to offer such training. The AAOS communication skills mentoring program, developed in collaboration with the Institute for Healthcare Communication in West Haven, Connecticut,[21] was initiated in 2001 after AAOS public opinion surveys revealed that the American public viewed orthopedic surgeons as "high tech, low touch."[22] These half-day communication skills workshops are very interactive, with only 20 percent of the time spent on didactic teaching. Orthopedic-specific video vignettes of medical interviews combined with role-playing, discussions, and feedback make up the majority of the workshop.[23]

John R. Tongue, MD, a practicing orthopedic surgeon in Tualatin, Oregon, and chair of the AAOS Communications Skills Project Team, has published an online list of patient encounter tips that are based on his interviews with more than 100,000 orthopedic patients and on the Institute for Healthcare Communication's Clinician-Patient Communication Course.[24] The AAOS has also pioneered the "Sign Your Site" program to reduce wrong-site surgical errors. Dr. Tongue has adapted the academy's recommendations as follows.

In my practice, my nurse, Jessie, simply tells every patient during the preoperative visit that I will be marking his or her surgery site. Then I mark the incision site itself and say, "I'll mark this more carefully in surgery." I place my initials on the patient's arm or leg. I think patients must feel a little strange being marked, so I sometimes say, "This is so they don't put you in the wrong room and take your gall bladder out!" They seem to really enjoy the comment, sometimes laughing loudly. Occasionally, if the patient seems nervous before my signing/marking, I'll say, "You know, there were a few famous orthopedic surgeons who didn't make it through their thirty-year careers keeping left and right straight! So I need to do this in my practice." Humility wins them over. My mark is made the day before the surgery, so I also reassure them that the mark will still be there after washing. And I look at all marks in the preop holding area immediately before surgery. I prefer to sign/mark in my office in advance as a way of educating the patient in a less stressful environment, but that won't work in all practice settings.

Patient can mark "yes" over my marks or "no" on the opposite side that won't be operated on. This does even more to assure them and the reviewing surgical team that we're all on the same page. Some patients might feel it isn't necessary to repeat the process, whereas others may think it's great (reassuring) to reconfirm the site.[25]

Active Listening

The ability to communicate effectively is vital to the practitioner-patient partnership. And how the practitioner says something can be even more important than what is actually said. The spoken words are important, but they aren't the only way in which messages are conveyed. It is estimated that as much as 93 percent of communication includes such nonverbal behaviors as tone of voice, mannerisms, and body language.[26] Caregivers who are proficient in active listening skills can greatly enhance the provider-patient relationship, as evidenced by the experiences of the patient mentioned earlier who was hospitalized for treatment of sepsis.

> Was the care I was receiving safe? My perceptions were influenced by staff member reactions to my questions and suggestions. Some technicians took the time to listen to me as I described the best site for a phlebotomy or how to position me so that my leg wound would be protected. I felt these staff members not only respected me but they also cared about my safety.

Listening effectively is hearing and understanding what the other person is saying. Health care providers must learn to be empathetic listeners, especially when the patient or family member is expressing a quality or safety concern. Chances are that many health care professionals have instinctively, or through practice, developed the skill of empathy; empathetic listening thus appears to be the easiest patient collaboration tool to learn. Yet this skill is often neglected in the hectic day-to-day delivery of health care services. And this oversight widens the gap between providers and patients, creating even greater safety concerns.

A University of Maine researcher, Dr. Marisue Pickering, identified four characteristics of empathetic listeners, as follows:

1. Desire to be other-directed rather than to project one's own feelings and ideas onto the other.

2. Desire to be nondefensive rather than to protect the self. When the self is being protected, it is difficult to focus on another person.

3. Desire to imagine the roles, perspectives, or experiences of the other rather than assuming they are the same as one's own.

4. Desire to listen as a receiver, not as a critic, and desire to understand the other person rather than to achieve either agreement from, or change in, that person.[27]

Some health care organizations are offering training sessions to help caregivers be more open and empathetic with patients. Skills taught in these training sessions include the following:

- Use of verbal and nonverbal communication to acknowledge input or questions from patients
- How to respond to the patient's verbal message through restating or paraphrasing
- Use of cues to reflect the patient's feelings, experiences, or statements
- How to offer tentative interpretations that reflect the patient's feelings, desires, or meanings
- Use of summarizing or synthesizing strategies to focus the feelings and/or concerns of patients
- How to respond when the patient requests more information or expresses confusion about some aspect of the health care experience
- How to support patients and families by showing warmth and caring
- How to check perceptions in a nondefensive manner to find out if the patient's interpretations and perceptions are valid and accurate
- How to give patients time to think as well as talk

George Bernard Shaw once wrote, "The greatest problem with communication is the illusion that it has been accomplished."

Communication is an essential part of the social contract between practitioners and patients. So when a patient and provider come together, building communication and collaboration can reduce poor outcomes and improve the patient's safety. As health care professionals come to appreciate the value and expertise of patients and families in reducing adverse events, the role of better communication will be evident. Communication is not just saying words; it is creating true understanding between caregivers and patients. Active listening is an important skill in that process.

Building Organizational Commitment

The organization acts as a host to the health care team, and as such, the manner in which the organization carries out the business of health service markedly affects the actions and attitudes of caregivers. Senior leaders determine overall purpose and policies and are responsible for decisions about how policies apply to physicians, nurses, and other members of the patient care team. The importance of partnering with patients and families to improve safety must be legitimized within the broader organization. A patient-centered culture of patient safety cannot be mandated administratively, nor can it be philosophically idealized into existence. Removing the division between patients and families on the one hand and providers on the other requires a fundamental shift in the culture of the organization. And culture change starts at the top.

Models for Culture Change

Experiences in changing the culture of safety at the Dana-Farber Cancer Institute (DFCI) in Boston have become a model for other organizations seeking to build better partnerships with patients and families. At DFCI, patients and families are treated as partners in care design, delivery, assessment, and improvement. Patients participate in the following arenas:

- Adult and pediatric patient and family advisory committees

- The adult oncology clinical services committee, during which discussion includes errors, falls, and other patient safety issues
- Facility planning
- Patient care rounds
- The patient educator program (cancer patients teach medical fellows about being a patient)
- The complementary therapy task force
- Friday meetings with the administrator[28]

Children's Hospitals and Clinics of Minnesota is another organization with a longtime commitment to involving patients and families in the health care experience. In 1999, the board of directors adopted quality and safety as an ethical obligation and the organization's number one shared value.[29] Through focused discussions with family members, the organization's senior leaders discovered what families already knew—patient care is risky and errors do occur. Families were looking for ways to be involved in safety improvement, and because the organization saw this as an opportunity to partner with patients and their families, it adopted a policy of open and honest communication with patients and families. The time, place, and circumstances of medical errors, as well as the consequences and actions taken to treat or ameliorate them, are shared. Senior leaders agreed that however bad the truth is, only one thing could be worse: never telling the truth and eliminating the opportunity for something to be done to prevent the mistake from happening again.

Julianne Morath, chief operating officer at Children's Hospitals and Clinics and 2002 winner of the John Eisenberg Award for Lifetime Achievement in Patient Safety, emphasizes that improved safety requires a partnership among members of the health care team and the patient and family members. In fact, says Morath, a culture of partnership is one of four important aspects of a safety culture. The other three aspects are an accountable culture, a just culture, and a culture of continuous learning.[30]

Patient and family partnerships are an important element in an organization's patient safety initiative. This component is clearly evident in the work being done at Murray-Calloway County Hospital in Murray, Kentucky. There is a clear top-down commitment to patient safety improvement (see figure 3-1).

Figure 3-1.   Organizational Safety Triangle at Murray-Calloway County Hospital

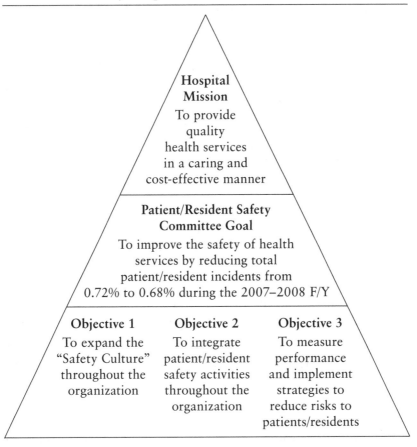

Source: Murray-Calloway County Hospital, Patient/Resident Safety Committee Goals and Objectives, 2007–2008. Reprinted with permission from Murray-Calloway County Hospital, Murray, Kentucky.

This commitment is articulated in many ways, such as the following:

- Multidisciplinary patient-resident safety committee, which includes physicians
- Patient safety integrated into the Leadership Plan for Provision of Patient Care
- Routine reporting from the patient-resident safety committee to the organization's leaders through the medical executive committee, quality council, and governing board using its Performance Improvement Priority Dashboard of patient safety issues
- Organizational shift in philosophy from punitive to "no blame" through implementation of the following:
  —Anonymous reporting option for medication errors (staff members who self-report receive a thank you note expressing appreciation for the employee's commitment to safety and for upholding the organization's value of honesty).
  —A copy of the note goes to the staff's director, who later uses the information as a positive element in the annual performance evaluation.
- Staff attendance required at patient safety-related training, including creation of a safety-conscious culture and patient partnership techniques
- Patient education provided through participation in a "Speak Up" campaign that covers all of the organization's entities: hospital, nursing home, home care, and hospice
- Staff participation in defining the "ABCs of Patient-Resident Safety" in the unique areas of the organization

The attitudes and beliefs of individual caregivers can greatly impact an organization's ability to create safety partnerships with patients and family members. Before embarking on a culture change initiative intended to increase patient involvement in safety, it is important to understand the prevailing culture. Ask caregivers to complete the self-assessment tool in figure 3-2 to

Figure 3-2.   Patient/Family Engagement Self-Assessment

Are you personally ready to engage patients and family in improving safety?

Instructions: Using the scale to the right, check the response that describes your level of agreement with each of the following items:	Strongly Disagree	Slightly Disagree	Neutral	Slightly Agree	Strongly Agree
1. I believe it is important to engage patients and families in preventing medical errors and adverse events.					
2. I believe that patient and family perspectives and opinions are as important as those of professionals.					
3. I believe that patients and families bring a safety viewpoint to the care team that no one else can provide.					
4. I consistently let patients/families know that I value their insights about safety.					
5. I work to create an environment in which patients and families feel supported and comfortable speaking up when they have concerns.					
6. I listen respectfully to the safety concerns of patients and their family members.					
7. I clearly state to patients and families what they can do to prevent medical errors and adverse events.					
8. I feel comfortable telling patients and families that caregivers might make a mistake or act unsafely.					
9. I feel comfortable asking patients and families to speak up if they think a caregiver has made a mistake or is acting unsafely.					
10. I know that all patients and family members cannot serve as safeguards in their care, and I do not place unrealistic expectations on individuals unable to participate in preventing medical errors and adverse events.					

determine how many of them are personally ready to engage patients and families in improving safety. Use the survey results to determine the willingness of caregivers to embrace patient and family involvement. If the level of willingness is low, don't start any large-scale patient partnership initiatives until you've spent some time educating caregivers on the value of such partnerships.

Demonstrating Commitment to the Patient

Nationwide attention is focused on the creation of health care provider "report cards" that allow consumers to make informed choices when selecting providers. Whether public access to comparative data on quality and outcomes will significantly affect consumer choice has yet to be determined. However, heightened media attention on patient safety has sensitized consumers to the realization that things can go wrong during the delivery of health care services.

Can a patient or family member determine whether a health care organization is truly committed to patient safety? The answer may not be apparent in a public report card about that organization's performance, but consumers most likely form an opinion about the safety of an organization through personal experiences and/or reports from those who have had personal experiences.[31] A recent study found that patients felt relatively safe while hospitalized, and ratings of safety correlated positively and highly with overall ratings of satisfaction with care.[32] Patients who were provided with more information about rights and safety-related topics at registration felt safer than those given less information.[33]

The Johns Hopkins Hospital in Baltimore, Maryland, demonstrates a commitment to patient involvement in safety efforts with its Patient Partnership Pledge (see figure 3-3). The pledge is posted on the Internet for all to see and distributed to patients and families in hard copy on admission. It is also posted on nursing units and in patient care/treatment rooms. The poster version is slightly different—there is space on the bottom for the unit manager to insert his or her name and contact number.

Figure 3-3. The Johns Hopkins Hospital Patient Partnership Pledge

Our Partnership Pledge

At Hopkins, we take a team approach to your safety.
We invite you and your family to join us as active
members of your care team.

We pledge to

- Coordinate your care
- Explain your care and treatment
- Listen to your questions or concerns
- Ask if you have safety concerns and take steps to address them.
- Ask about your pain often and keep you as comfortable as possible
- Check your identification before any medication, treatment or procedure
- Label all lab samples in your presence
- Clean our hands often

We ask you, or a loved one, to

- Ask questions
- Speak up if you are concerned about a test, procedure or medicine
- Check the information on your ID bracelet for accuracy
- Be clear and complete about your medical history, including current medications
- Clean your hands often and remind your visitors to do the same
- Remind us if we do not carry out our pledge to you

We welcome your involvement and feedback. The unit manager is available to hear
concerns about your care and safety.

From the doctors, nurses and staff of The Johns Hopkins Hospital

Source: Johns Hopkins Hospital, Baltimore, Maryland. Used with permission.

Even though patients and their families may be uninformed in matters of technical or clinical performance, they are often able to discern an organization's commitment to safety through the attitudes and actions of caregivers. The experiences of the patient who was hospitalized for treatment of sepsis illustrate the consumer's perspective.

The view from the bedside is a trusting position until expectations run amuck. The patient's capacity to hear all the discussion over many shifts creates a sense of inconsistency. There is fear that a thin thread is holding the treatment together, and perhaps the unthinkable will happen and the patient will become a victim.

As time passes in my hospital stay, a familiar routine emerges. Running the antibiotic through the line takes one hour. The antibiotic drip needs to start by a certain time so that other treatments, such as my trip to physical therapy, can be under way by 10 in the morning. This sounds simple, but inefficiencies and the possibility of breaking the thread of safety abound.

What if the antibiotic is started just half an hour late? The treatment might not be finished by the time I go to the physical therapy department for a whirlpool treatment on my leg wound. The facility has only one whirlpool, lots of people in the hospital need treatments, and the physical therapy department has a tight schedule. What if I miss my scheduled whirlpool treatment time because the antibiotic hasn't finished infusing? Or if I go to physical therapy with the IV still running, will a nurse leave the floor and find me to flush the line when the antibiotic has finished running in? I was told that flushing the line is important; otherwise, I might lose critical access. Then what?

Issues that seemed inconsequential to me when I was the bedside nurse have taken on a whole different meaning now that I am a patient. When I share my fears with staff members, they seem to brush me off. One of the wheels on the IV pole is broken and won't swivel and is why I need a nurse to help me go to the bathroom when the IV is running in. It takes an average of $14\frac{1}{2}$ minutes for a nurse to answer my call light. My bladder seldom lasts that long. I wonder if other, more important aspects of my treatment will go any better?

Organizations committed to patient safety do more than hand out pamphlets to inform patients that "It's okay to ask questions and to expect answers you understand." Personal safety is a common concern for all patients, yet for a variety of reasons many don't speak up when they are fearful of caregivers making a mistake. That's why organizations committed to patient safety are proactive in partnering with patients and family members. Everyone must be willing to admit that mistakes can happen and be up front in explaining to patients what is being done to reduce the chance of errors (including what the patient can do). The more often that patients can be made to feel in control of a seemingly out-of-control situation, the greater will be their sense of safety and camaraderie with the health care team. As patients' feelings of control rise, so will their willingness to speak up when something doesn't seem to be going just right.

Empower Patients with Information

Whose responsibility is it to educate patients about their role in patient safety? Since the 1999 release of the Institute of Medicine's report *To Err Is Human,* a number of national and state governmental agencies and organizations have undertaken initiatives aimed at educating consumers about their role in health care safety and error prevention. "Be Involved in Your Health Care: Tips to Help Prevent Medical Errors," published by the Virginians Improving Patient Care and Safety in Richmond, Virginia, is just one of the many pamphlets and fact sheets that have been created at the state level to enlighten consumers.[34]

Community outreach activities are taking place throughout the country. For example, the Madison (WI) Patient Safety Collaborative has sponsored public events at senior centers throughout the city to promote medication safety and fall prevention and reduction.[35] The Partnering for Patient Empowerment through Community Awareness (PPECA) project, a collaboration among patient safety advocates, health sciences librarians, health care institutions, and public libraries, has held several informational sessions at public libraries throughout northern Illinois to educate consumers on patient safety issues.[36] The PPECA has developed training tools for libraries and health care organizations interested in offering similar sessions in local communities.[37]

Nationally, groups such as the Agency for Healthcare Research and Quality[38] and the Institute for Safe Medication Practices[39] have published numerous resources on what consumers can do to reduce medication errors and prevent untoward outcomes. The

Joint Commission has made its Speak Up brochures available to the public as well as to health care organizations.[40]

Consumer groups are also very much involved in getting the word out. For example, PULSE America, a not-for-profit organization, is working to reduce the rate of medical errors by educating the public and advocating a safer health care system.[41] The acronym PULSE stands for Persons United Limiting Substandards and Errors in Health Care. The not-for-profit group Parents of Infants and Children with Kernicterus has worked to educate health care professionals and the public about the dangers of severe newborn jaundice with the goal of preventing kernicterus, a condition that causes severe cerebral palsy.[42] The Institute for Family-Centered Care[43] offers consumers a unique look at how to become safety partners with caregivers to improve quality.

Patients as Safety Partners

The patient safety educational strategies for consumers are reminiscent of the initiatives undertaken in the early 1990s to familiarize the public with clinical practice guidelines. Developers of these guidelines created consumer-friendly versions for distribution to the public, and various groups incorporated guideline recommendations into patient teaching materials. Creating informed patients was considered an important strategy for improving practitioner compliance with the guidelines and reducing unnecessary costs associated with inappropriate care.[44] This strategy of creating informed patients continues today, with numerous mass information campaigns and consumer-directed education opportunities sponsored by payers, health care providers, and consumer groups. Now, more than ten years after the concept of empowering patients with information was first introduced on a national level, many consumers have become informed and proactive in health care decision making.

The empowerment of patients to become partners in the patient safety movement is a logical extension of the consumer education initiatives started in the 1990s. Lessons learned during the earlier guideline education campaigns should be applied to the safety movement. One important feature of successful public education strategies is diversity. Education can be:

- Informal or formal
- Impersonal or personal
- One way or interactive
- Isolated or connected to ongoing relationships
- Knowledge oriented or change oriented[45]

Already a number of practices and resources are aimed at encouraging patients to share responsibility for their own safety.[46] Although these initiatives are valuable, getting the message to individual consumers will require one-on-one interactions with health care providers. Research on the impact of different physician education strategies for implementing guidelines has indicated that personal, interactive strategies tended to be more influential in changing practitioner behavior than have more formal or indirect approaches.[47] This is an important lesson for those seeking to empower consumers with the knowledge to become more involved in health care safety.

The economist Joseph Schumpeter wrote in 1939 that "it was not enough to produce satisfactory soap, it was also necessary to induce people to wash."[48] This sentiment was echoed by John Williamson in a 1991 contribution to a book from the American College of Physician Executives. Here Williamson emphasized that physicians needed to be educated on the importance of providing better information to patients about various treatment options and expected outcomes.[49] Similar practitioner education must occur as it relates to patient safety information.

Every contact between caregivers and consumers must be seen as an opportunity to disseminate information about the patient's role in safety. Physicians, nurses, and other caregivers must personally interact with patients and family members to impart information. Mass education campaigns will only be successful if the message is consistently reinforced at the patient-caregiver level. Several health care organizations have already begun to initiate one-on-one patient safety dialogues between caregivers and patients. Some examples of these efforts follow.

Partnership Initiatives That Work

Partnering with patients has been a vital component of patient safety at the University of Wisconsin (UW) Hospital and Clinics in Madison for several years. The organization uses many different strategies to communicate the patient safety message to the public. One of the first projects, done in conjunction with the Madison Patient Safety Collaborative, was developing a consumer brochure called "Using Your Medications Safely: A Guide to Prescription Health."[50] This colorful eight-page pamphlet covers such topics as the following:

- Questions to ask your health care provider and pharmacist
- How to make the most of your visit to your health care provider
- How to make the most of your trip to the pharmacy
- Optimizing your medication use at home
- Maximizing medication safety when you are in the hospital
- Considerations for selecting a pharmacy

A medication wallet card is included in the brochure, as are instructions for using it effectively. The brochure is distributed to all patients at the time of hospital admission and used for education purposes by pharmacists and other caregivers. It is also available in all the clinic areas.

At the UW Hospital and Clinics, patients and families are very involved in medication reconciliation on admission and in learning about their medications on discharge. Each patient receives a medication interview from a pharmacist when admitted. If the patient is unable to communicate at the time of admission and family is not available, pharmacists routinely contact other sources (local pharmacies, physician offices, nursing homes, and so forth) to obtain information on medication use. At the time of discharge, a pharmacist provides medication teaching to the patient.

The UW Hospital and Clinics has also assembled an extensive library of patient education materials. Included in this library are fact sheets and brochures containing information on the role of patients and family members in making health care safer, such as the following:

- CT scans and safety
- Using restraints safely, and why restraint use is limited as much as possible
- How to prevent falls

All patient education materials are reviewed and revised as needed at least every three years.

Posted in each patient room at the UW Hospital are tips on safety for patients and family members. In addition, caregivers encourage patients and their family to contact the patient relations department about any concerns, including matters related to patient safety. Feedback is used by the organization to make changes as appropriate. At the UW Children's Hospital, parent and adolescent advisory groups were formed several years ago to provide input into patient care issues, including safety. The advisory group concept has now been extended to the adult population at the UW Hospital to ensure that patients and families are provided opportunities to proactively improve patient safety.

It is important to gain feedback from staff during the development of patient and family collaboration initiatives. At Presbyterian Healthcare in Charlotte, North Carolina, a draft list of suggested safety partnership practices to be distributed to patients and families was circulated among staff for input. Every group who examined the list offered some insight into how patient safety practices are actually used by caregivers. For example, staff noted that patients often wonder why they are repeatedly asked their name and date of birth. So the script was redesigned to let patients know that this questioning was a way for staff to engage them in safety management. The patient should expect every provider to ask these questions. Furthermore, patients are encouraged to ask for clarification to fully understand each step of their care.

The finalized list (see figure 3-4) was approved by senior operations, the medical board, and the unit clinical coordinators. In addition to providing the list in hard copy to outpatients and hospital admissions, a video slide show was developed for patient and family viewing on the hospital's closed-circuit televisions and on DVD players in the outpatient areas. The patient safety video is also used to orient new staff to the organization's patient safety culture.

Highline Medical Center in Burien, Washington, has developed a unique "Care Partner" program in which a volunteer family member or other partner, at the request of the patient, is trained to be a participant in the care process.[51] Care partners are shown where various comfort aids (e.g., blankets, water) are located and are encouraged to use them. Care partners may participate in dressing changes, keep track of medications and diagnostic tests, ask questions on the patient's behalf, become familiar with the various physicians and other caregivers on the unit, and play a role in reporting on the patient's condition. Care partners assist the nurses by being the "eyes and ears" of the nurse, providing touches that only a family member can offer, and ensuring that a patient's concerns are voiced in a timely manner.

A number of health care organizations are expanding opportunities for patients and family members to serve on patient safety advisory groups. The traditional role of consumer advisory groups has been to suggest environmental or "cosmetic"

Figure 3-4. Presbyterian Healthcare Safety Orientation for Patients and Families, Charlotte, North Carolina

Good day, and welcome to our remarkable hospital. We thank you and your physician for choosing us for your healthcare needs. Together, with your physician, we strive to make your hospital experience the best by providing excellent care. The following information is designed to help prepare you for your hospital stay and your recovery. Working with you, our goal is that you will have an excellent experience at Presbyterian Healthcare.

We are all here for your safety and to assist you in your healing process. During your time with us, please understand that your safety is one of our main concerns. We ask that you also make safety a priority. You can help us by following these safety rules.

1. If you cannot speak for yourself, or your illness leaves you drowsy, we suggest that you have someone with you to help with these safety rules. It is important for you to be involved in your healthcare decisions. We offer communication aids such as interpreters to assist with language at no charge to you. Ask questions about your condition and care. Make sure you get results of any tests or procedures. Ask if you have not heard.

2. As our staff care for you, you will be repeatedly asked your name and date of birth. We do this on purpose to match the right person with the right treatment.

3. We will ask you what medicines you are currently taking. Provide a complete and accurate list for us. We write these medicines in your medical chart.

4. Let us know if you have any allergies. We are most interested and need to know about allergies to medicines, foods, and latex. Latex is found in items such as gloves. We will tell all healthcare providers if you have any allergies by recording a note in your medical chart.

5. Ask the name of the medicine and ask why you are being given this medicine.

6. It is important that all healthcare providers clean their hands before touching you. You can observe our staff or ask them if they have cleaned their hands.

7. If you have a surgical procedure that could be done on the left or right, such as with arm surgery, you will be asked to mark your surgery site with a "yes".

(Continued on next page)

Figure 3-4.   (Continued)

8. If you have any increased pain or discomfort even if it does not relate to why you are in the hospital, please tell someone right away.

9. If you have a PCA pump to help manage your pain, you, the patient, should be the only one to press the button that gives you a prescribed dose of pain medicine.

10. Do not adjust any medical equipment. If the equipment alarms, use your call bell to call for assistance.

11. Call for assistance when getting out of bed, especially if you are starting a new medicine.

We are very pleased you and your doctor have chosen Presbyterian Healthcare for your medical care. We hope this video has helped prepare you for your hospital stay. If you have any questions regarding this information, please ask your nurse or other healthcare provider. Our goal is for you to have an excellent experience with us. Please let us know if there is anything before, during, or after your stay that we can do for you.

Source: Presbyterian Healthcare, Charlotte, North Carolina. 2007. Used with permission.

changes such as expansion of parking areas or more comfortable waiting areas. In a safety advisory capacity, former patients and family members are partnering with caregivers to reduce adverse events or system breakdowns that are potentially harmful. The behavioral health department at Mount Sinai Hospital in New York City formed an advisory council composed of staff and family members for the purpose of improving the patient discharge process.[52] Family members often shoulder the responsibility of ensuring their loved one gets needed medication and treatment after leaving the hospital. The stories shared by the family members of the advisory council alerted staff to problems that might not otherwise have been recognized. For instance, family members felt they got left "holding the bag" after the patient's discharge. In response, Mount Sinai has established a navigator role to assist families in helping patients get needed medications and follow-up treatment. The partnership between staff and family members at the advisory council has been energizing for everyone involved, and, most importantly, the safety of patient care has been improved.

The adult patient and family advisory council created at Vanderbilt University Hospital in Nashville, Tennessee, includes one patient who had a heart transplant, two patients with diabetes, and a woman whose husband died at the hospital from burns sustained in a plane crash.[53] Input from these consumers has resulted in several patient safety improvements. For example, reclining chairs with longer leg rests were purchased for the treatment rooms after it was learned from the diabetic patients that the current chairs impeded circulation in their legs.

Engagement of patients and family members is expanding to the bedside and challenging the traditional paternalistic role of caregivers. A common complaint of patients and their family members is that physicians and other staff don't listen to their concerns.[54] Yet, often these concerns are well founded. Consider the event below reported by the Pennsylvania Patient Safety Authority.

A patient told a lab tech not to draw blood from the right arm, but blood was drawn from that arm anyway. There was an order not to use that arm because it was to be used for a dialysis shunt. The patient also was wearing a color-coded bracelet indicating that the arm should not be used for blood draws.[55]

In some health care organizations the patient described above would have a formal means to speak up and be heard. University of Pittsburgh Medical Center (UPMC) Shadyside Hospital, a 486-bed affiliate of the UPMC, was one of the first organizations to implement a response team that could be initiated by patients and families.[56] The initiative, entitled Condition Help (shortened to Condition H), empowers patients or family members to call a number on the hospital phone to deploy a rapid response team, which arrives at the patient's location within a few minutes. The team consists of a representative from the patient relations department, the administrative nursing coordinator on duty, one physician, and staff from the patient's location.[57] In the first thirteen months following the start of the initiative in July 2005, Condition H was called thirty-eight times by patients or family members, with an average of 2.9 calls per month. "More than half of these calls potentially prevented a more serious clinical problem," according to Beth Kuzminsky, RN, MSN, staff associate for the Center for Quality Improvement and Innovation at UPMC.[58]

Today, several more hospitals have adopted similar rapid response strategies. In 2006, Carolinas Medical Center–NorthEast (CMC-NE) in Concord, North Carolina, expanded its clinician-activated response team initiative to allow patients or family members to activate the teams. The CMC-NE initiative is called Code Care.[59] An important component of patient-activated response teams is education. Carolinas Medical Center–NorthEast distributes its Code Care pamphlet (see figure 3-5) to patients and family members, and a tent card with similar information is placed at the patient's bedside. Staff education is equally important. A two-page brochure (see figure 3-6) is used to educate CMC-NE staff to the Code Care purpose and process. To further strengthen patient-caregiver communication, CMC-NE has created scripted responses for the Code Care team and staff (see figure 3-7).

An Aspiration, Not a Project

Organizations that have developed successful safety partnerships with patients and family members have one factor in common—the initiatives are not treated as projects with defined start and stop dates. Rather, the organizations aspire to continually seek out new and innovative ways of engaging consumers in the safety improvement journey. And everyone in the organization, from the board of directors to the frontline caregivers, has a role in realizing success. Is your organization committed to patient/family safety partnerships? The checklist in figure 3-8 provides an organizational blueprint for success. Use this checklist to identify and correct shortcomings.

Figure 3-5.   *Code Care* **Informational Brochure for Patients and Families, Carolinas Medical Center–NorthEast, Concord, North Carolina**

Code Care, Rapid Response Team

Carolinas Medical Center–NorthEast is dedicated to making the hospital a safe place for patient care to happen.

As a response to providing the best care to our patients, we created a *Code Care response.*

Code Care was created to address the needs of the patient in the case of an emergency or when the patient is unable to get the attention of a health care provider. This call will provide our patients and families an avenue to call for immediate help when they feel they are not receiving adequate medical attention in an emergent situation.

When to call

- If a noticeable medical change in the patient occurs that needs immediate attention and the health care team is not recognizing the concern.

- If there is a breakdown in how care is being given and/or confusion over what needs to be done for the patient in an emergent situation.

To access Code Care, please call 8888 from a hospital phone. The operator will ask for caller identification, room number, patient name and patient concern. The operator will immediately activate a "Code Care" where a team of medical professionals are alerted and will arrive in the room to assess the situation. Additional clinical supports will be called in as needed.

In offering our families the Code Care option, we want you to know that you are our partners in care. If you have any questions, please discuss them with one of our health care providers.

Source: Carolinas Medical Center–NorthEast, Concord, North Carolina. 2007. Used with permission.

Figure 3-6.   *CodeCare* Staff Education Brochure, Carolinas Medical Center–NorthEast, Concord, North Carolina

---

Code Care—A Help Line for Patients and Families

We believe that *teamwork* is the best way to provide safe care to our patients. As Carolinas Medical Center–NorthEast grows to become a hospital of the future, we ask that our patients, families, and visitors become part of the *team* to provide the safest care possible. **Code Care** is all about *teamwork.*

What Is Code Care?

Code Care is a telephone *help line* that patients and families can call if they notice a serious change in their condition but have been unable to contact a caregiver on the unit or feel unable to express their concern during what they perceive as an urgent situation.

Code Care should be called:

• When there is confusion over what needs to be done for the patient,

• If there are care conflicts between patient/family and caregivers,

• When there is a breakdown in communication, or

• When there is an urgent need for patient care in a serious situation.

Code Care is All about Saving Lives:

The idea of **Code Care** started after an 18 month old little girl named Josie King died in one of our country's best hospitals due to a breakdown in communication between her family and her caregivers. Since this tragedy, Josie's mother, Sorrel King, has worked with hospitals and the Institute for Healthcare Improvement (IHI) to promote **Code Care** across the country.

How Will Code Care be Called?

Patients and families should first be told about **Code Care** when they are admitted to the hospital.

Use the following script to tell your patients and families about Code Care:

> *"If you ever feel like you are not getting the care you or your loved one need and the situation is an emergency, then you can call Code Care by dialing 8888 on any phone in the hospital where the patient is located. The hospital operator will ask you where you are located, the patient's name, and the reason for the call. Within minutes, a small team of caregivers will arrive to help you."*

Figure 3-6.   (Continued)

Who will respond to a Code Care?

An ICU Nurse, the Nursing Supervisor, a patient representative from the Share the Care team, and a Respiratory Therapist will respond to calls, but will check-in with the primary nurse or charge nurse BEFORE going to the patient.

Carolinas Medical Center–NorthEast is one of the first hospitals in the country to provide **Code Care** for our patients and families in response to the King family's tragic loss. Everyone's help is needed to make **Code Care** a success as we continue to be committed to providing patients, families and visitors the safest, quality care possible.

Source: Carolinas Medical Center–NorthEast, Concord, North Carolina. 2007. Used with permission.

Figure 3-7.   *CodeCare* Scripting for Staff at Carolinas Medical Center–NorthEast, Concord, North Carolina

• Script for Code Care team when arriving on the unit and approaching unit staff/charge nurse:

> *"Hello, my name is _____. I need to let you know that a Code Care was called from the patient/family in _____ room/location."*

If the staff/charge nurse is NOT aware of the situation, then respond by saying:

> *"Let's go find out what's going on with the patient/family together."*

If the staff/charge nurse IS aware of the situation, then respond by saying:

> *"What can I do to help you with the situation?"*

• Script for Code Care team or unit staff approaching the patient/family:

Entering patient's room:

> *"Hello, my name is _____ from the Code Care team—Thank you for calling us. What can we do to help you?"*

Departing:

> *"Thank you. Is there anything else I/we can do for you?"*

• Script for Code Care team when departing the unit and staff:

> *"What can I do to assist you before I go? Thanks again for your help."*

Source: Carolinas Medical Center–NorthEast, Concord, North Carolina. 2007. Used with permission.

**Figure 3-8.   Creating Safety Partnerships with Patients—
            An Organizational Blueprint**

☐ Identify clear strategic aims and objectives. What do you want to achieve?

☐ Communicate your strategic aims and objectives to everyone in the organization. Does everyone understand what you are trying to achieve?

☐ Earmark a budget for patient/family safety partnership initiatives. Do you have the time and resources to involve all stakeholders effectively?

☐ Involve stakeholders appropriate to your aims and objectives. Are you involving the range of caregivers, support staff, and consumers most likely to be affected?

☐ With input from all stakeholders, develop specific tactics to achieve your aims and objectives. Do you have a multiplicity of strategies?

☐ Identify the anticipated role of caregivers and support staff. Is everyone clear about the purpose of patient/family safety partnerships and their role?

☐ Provide training. Do physicians/staff have the skills, confidence, and credibility to effectively engage patients and families as safety partners?

☐ Provide education and support for patients/families. Do patients and families have ready access to safety partnership advice and support?

☐ Keep people informed about what is being done to create patient/family safety partnerships. What is happening as a result of your efforts? Are you celebrating successes?

☐ Evaluate the impact of patient/family safety partnerships on the processes and outcomes of health care services. What things are working well? What needs to be changed? Did the partnerships make a difference?

Being Safe Together

Your Majesty, please . . . I don't like to complain,
But down here below, we are feeling great pain.
I know, up on top you are seeing great sights,
But down at the bottom, we, too, should have rights.
—Theodore "Dr. Seuss" Geisel (Yertle the Turtle)

There is overwhelming evidence that the safety of health care services can be improved. Although health care providers bear the major responsibility for reducing unintended medical errors, consumers can and should be encouraged to speak up for their own safety. And when patients and family members do speak up, providers must openly acknowledge and value their input.

Currently there is only anecdotal evidence that practitioner-patient partnerships can reduce adverse events, but common sense suggests that adding another safeguard—the patient—will not make matters worse. Some patients, fed up with what appears to be a national epidemic of medical misadventures, are demanding they be viewed as error prevention participants.

Consider the hindsight perspective of the nurse turned hospital patient for treatment of sepsis.

I was told that I would be discharged when the CT scan results had been called to the physician's office. There was a one-and-a-half-day administrative delay from the time of the physician's order for the CT scan until it was actually completed. When I returned from radiology, I got dressed in my street clothes and stood at the nurse's station waiting for my discharge instructions. One nurse looked at me and said, "Why are you dressed?" No one knew I was to go home that day.

An error that health care professionals have made over and over again is to think they know what the patient wants, feels, needs. However, we don't know and we can't know until we've been there. My experiences as a hospital patient made me realize that many health care professionals (including myself) lack the skills or desire needed to effectively partner with patients. Just

a simple explanation of what to expect during my hospitalization, offered as soon as possible after my admission, would have
reduced my anxieties. I wouldn't have been so quick to assume
that things were going wrong, and I would have known when to
speak up with valid concerns. Instead, I became the patient every
health care professional dreads—constantly asking questions
and seemingly never satisfied with the answers. By listening and
learning from patients and their family members, we can realize
significant safety improvements. The collaboration strategies and
tools need not be expensive or difficult; they need only be used.

Health care providers and practitioners can create stronger partnerships with patients by building on past health care
consumer education initiatives. This can be accomplished by
validating that mistakes do occur in the delivery of health care
services and then helping patients and families regain control
(and self-esteem). Patients must be taught how to help themselves as they navigate the confusing and sometimes treacherous health care delivery system. In many instances, the patient
is the only constant thread throughout the continuum of care.
The patient's persistent and informed vigilance is a critical
aspect of patient safety.

Most health care organizations have some components
of patient safety already in place, and a few are aggressively
involving patients and family members in error reduction activities. Health care organizations often have to overcome cultural
barriers and outmoded attitudes before an outreach to patients
and families can be successful. Once the patient safety mind-
set begins to take hold in the organization, it's time to create
opportunities for consumer involvement in the patient safety
movement. The most important consideration is that organizations start somewhere—whether it's staff training in active
listening skills or creation of patient-activated rapid response
teams. Partnering with consumers to improve the safety of
health care services is not an event; it is a journey—a journey
well worth taking.

References

1. A. Gawande, *Complications: A Surgeon's Notes on an Imperfect Science* (New York: Metropolitan Books, 2002).
2. C. Perrow, *Normal Accidents: Living with High-Risk Technologies* (New York: Basic Books, 1984), 89–100.
3. American Hospital Association, "Improving Medication Safety by Partnering with Patients," Quality Advisory (September 15, 2000).
4. Joint Commission, "Speak Up" Campaign, March 2002 (Oakbrook Terrace, IL: Joint Commission) [http://www.jcaho.org/general+public/patient+safety/speak+up/speak+up.htm].
5. National Patient Safety Foundation, Chicago [http://www.npsf.org/download/PreventingInfections.pdf]. Accessed October 2007.
6. Agency for Healthcare Research and Quality, "AHRQ and National Council on Patient Information and Education Produce New Tool to Help Consumers Reduce Medication Errors," April 30, 2003 (press release) (Rockville, MD: AHRQ) [http://www.ahcpr.gov/news/press/pr2003/safemedpr.htm]. Accessed December 11, 2007.
7. A. D. Waterman, T. H. Gallagher, J. Garbutt, B. M. Waterman, V. Fraser, and T. E. Burroughs, "Brief Report: Hospitalized Patients' Attitudes about and Participation in Error Prevention," *Journal of General Internal Medicine* 21, no. 4 (2006): 367–70.
8. A. J. Kuzel, S. H. Woolf, V. J. Gilchrist, J. D. Engel, T. A. LaVeist, C. Vincent, and R. M. Frankel, "Patient Reports of Preventable Problems and Harms in Primary Health Care," *Annals of Family Medicine* 2, no. 4 (2004): 333–40.
9. C. W. DiGiovanni, L. Kang, and J. Manuel, "Patient Compliance in Avoiding Wrong-Site Surgery," *Journal of Bone and Joint Surgery* (American) 85, no. 5 (2003): 815–19.
10. T. Bodenheimer, E. H. Wagner, and K. Grumbach, "Improving Primary Care for Patients with Chronic Illness," *Journal of the American Medical Association* 288, no. 14 (2002): 1775–79.
11. L. T. Kohn, J. M. Corrigan, and M. S. Donaldson, eds., *To Err Is Human: Building a Safer Health System*, Institute of Medicine Committee on Quality of Health Care in America (Washington, DC: National Academies Press, 1999), 150.
12. American College of Physicians, "The Role of the Patient in Patient Safety" (Tampa, FL: ACPE) [http://www.acponline.org/ptsafety/patient.htm]. Accessed October 2007.
13. National Patient Safety Foundation, "National Agenda for Action: Patients and Families in Patient Safety: Nothing About Me, Without Me" (Chicago: National Patient Safety Foundation, 2003) [http://www.npsf.org/download/AgendaFamilies.pdf]. Accessed October 2007.

14. Joint Commission, "FAQs for the Joint Commission's 2007 National Patient Safety Goals" (Oakbrook Terrace, IL: Joint Commission) [http://www.jointcommission.org/NR/rdonlyres/4EDAB705-F663-4D29-9449-EC0191063BD0/0/07_NPSG_FAQs_13.pdf]. Accessed October 2007.

15. C. Edwards, "A Proposal That Patients Be Considered Honorary Members of the Healthcare Team," *Journal of Clinical Nursing* 11, no. 3 (2002): 340–48.

16. N. K. G Mendis, ed., *The Questions of King Milinda: Abr't of Milindapanha* (Seattle: Pariyatti Press, 1993).

17. M. A. LaCombe, "On Bedside Teaching," *Annals of Internal Medicine* 126, no. 3 (1997): 217–20.

18. M. E. Knowles, *The Modern Practice of Adult Education* (Englewood Cliffs, NJ: Cambridge/Prentice Hall, 1980), 43–44.

19. B. Nair, J. Coughlan, and M. Hensley, "Student and Patient Perspectives on Bedside Teaching," *Medical Education* 31, no. 5 (1997): 341–46.

20. P. N. Uhlig and colleagues, "Reconfiguring Clinical Teamwork for Safety and Effectiveness," *Focus on Patient Safety* 5, no. 3 (2002): 1–2.

21. Institute for Healthcare Communication, West Haven, CT [http://www.healthcarecomm.org]. Accessed February 2008.

22. American Academy of Orthopaedic Surgeons, *1999 Public Image Investigation. Second Report* (Rosemont, IL: American Academy of Orthopaedic Surgeons, 1999).

23. American Academy of Orthopaedic Surgeons, Communication Skills Mentoring Program [http://www3.aaos.org/education/csmp/index.cfm]. Accessed October 2007.

24. J. R. Tongue, "Patient Encounter Tips," AAOS Communication Skills Mentoring Program [http://www3.aaos.org/education/csmp/PatientEncounterTips.cfm]. Accessed October 2007.

25. Personal correspondence between Patrice Spath and Dr. John Tongue, May 26, 2003.

26. A. Mehrabian, *Silent Messages* (Belmont, CA: Wadsworth, 1971).

27. M. Pickering, "Communication," *Explorations: A Journal of Research of the University of Maine* 3, no. 1 (1986): 16–19.

28. James Conway, "Tools for Patient Safety," conference presentation, Beyond State Reporting: Medical Errors and Patient Safety Issues, Nashville, TN, June 6–8, 2001.

29. G. Sprenger, "Deal to Tell It All," conference presentation, 3rd Annenberg Conference on Patient Safety, St. Paul, MN, 2001.

30. J. Morath, "Changing the Culture of Patient Safety," conference presentation, BJC HealthCare Patient Safety Forum, St. Louis, MO, 2003.

31. K. Davis, S. C. Schoenbaum, K. S. Collins, K. Tenney, D. L. Hughes, and A.-M. J. Audet, *Room for Improvement: Patient Reports on the*

Quality of Their Health Care (New York: Commonwealth Fund, 2002).

32. R. J. Wolosin, L. Vercler, and J. L. Matthews, "Am I Safe Here? Improving Patients' Perceptions of Safety in Hospitals," *Journal of Nursing Care Quality* 21, no. 1 (2006): 30–38.

33. Ibid.

34. Virginians Improving Patient Care and Safety, "Be Involved in Your Health Care: Tips to Help Prevent Medical Errors," Richmond, VA [http://www.vipcs.org]. Accessed October 2007.

35. Madison Patient Safety Collaborative, "Patient Falls Initiative" (Madison, WI: MPSC) [http://www.madisonpatientsafety.org/index.htm]. Accessed October 2007.

36. L. Zipperer, M. Berendsen, and L. Walton, "Empowering Patients at the Public Library," *Patient Safety and Quality Healthcare* (March/April 2006) [http://www.psqh.com/marapr06/consumers.html]. Accessed October 2007.

37. Partnering for Patient Empowerment through Community Awareness [http://www.galter.northwestern.edu/ppeca/]. The site includes speaker templates, reading lists, examples of handouts for distribution at each session, and a facilitator's guide.

38. Agency for Healthcare Research and Quality, "Consumers & Patients" (Rockville, MD: AHRQ) [http://www.ahrq.gov/consumer/]. Accessed February 2008.

39. Institute for Safe Medication Practices, "Consumers Can Prevent Medication Errors" (Huntingdon Valley, PA) [http://www.ismp.org/consumers]. Accessed February 2008.

40. Joint Commission, "Speak Up" (Oakbrook Terrace, IL: Joint Commission, 2007) [http://www.jointcommission.org/GeneralPublic/Speak+Up/]. Accessed October 2007.

41. PULSE America (New York) [http://www.pulseamerica.org]. Accessed February 2008)

42. Parents of Infants and Children with Kernicterus (Chicago) [http://www.pickonline.org]. Accessed February 2008.

43. Institute for Family-Centered Care (Bethesda, MD) [http://www.familycenteredcare.org]. Accessed February 2008.

44. M. J. Field and K. N. Lohr, eds., *Guidelines for Clinical Practice: From Development to Use,* Committee on Clinical Practice Guidelines, Institute of Medicine (Washington, DC: National Academies Press, 1992), 83–88.

45. Ibid., 88.

46. L. T. Pizzi, N. I. Goldfarb, and D. B. Nash, "Other Practices Related to Patient Participation," in *Making Health Care Safer: A Critical Analysis of Patient Safety Practices,* AHRQ Publication 01-E058 (Rockville, MD: Agency for Healthcare Research and Quality, U.S. Department of Health and Human Services, July 20, 2001).

47. Field and Lohr, *Guidelines for Clinical Practice,* 88.
48. J. Schumpeter, *Business Cycles: A Theoretical, Historical, and Statistical Analysis of the Capitalist Press* (New York: McGraw-Hill, 1939).
49. J. Williamson, "Medical Quality Management Systems in Perspective," in *Health Care Quality Management for the 21st Century,* ed. J. Couch (Tampa, FL: American College of Physician Executives, 1991).
50. This brochure is available to download on the Web site of the Madison Patient Safety Collaborative [http://www.madisonpatientsafety.org].
51. ECRI Institute, "JCAHO [Joint Commission] Proposal for Patient-Centered Care Brings Concept to Mainstream Healthcare Settings," *Risk Management Reporter* 24, no. 3 (2005): 1–7.
52. Karen Bry and Robin Czaijka, "Mount Sinai Hospital Inpatient Psychiatric Family Advisory Council," conference presentation, Illinois Hospital Association 3rd Annual Safety Connections Conference, Bloomington, IL, October 24, 2007.
53. Laura Landro, "Hospitals Boost Patients' Power as Advisers," *Wall Street Journal,* August 8, 2007, D-1.
54. Patrice Spath, "Safety from the Patient's Point of View," in *Partnering with Patients to Reduce Medical Errors,* P. L. Spath, ed. (Chicago: Health Forum, 2004).
55. Pennsylvania Patient Safety Authority, "When Patients Speak—Collaboration in Patient Safety," *Patient Safety Advisory* 2, no. 1 (2005): 1 [http://www.psa.state.pa.us/psa/lib/psa/advisories/v2n1march2005/vol_2-1-march-05-article_a-patients_speak.pdf]. Accessed October 2007. Used with permission.
56. P. K. Greenhouse, B. Kuzminsky, S. C. Martin, and T. Merryman, "Calling a Condition H(elp)," *American Journal of Nursing* 106, no. 11 (2006): 63–66.
57. P. L. Spath, "Empowering Families in Emergencies," *Hospitals & Health Networks OnLine* (first appeared February 20, 2007) [http://www.hhnmag.com/hhnmag_app/jsp/articledisplay.jsp?dcrpath=HHNMAG/Article/data/02FEB2007/0702HHN_Online_Spath&domain=HHNMAG]. Accessed December 12, 2007.
58. Ibid.
59. Ibid.

4

Engaging Patients in Safety: Barriers and Solutions

Michelle H. Pelling

Health care consumers have a legitimate interest in their own safety. For this reason, many patients are becoming acculturated to the need for actively participating in their own care. At most stages of health care, there is the potential for patients to contribute to their own care through the provision of pertinent health information, participation in the plan of care and treatment decisions, and self-management of their condition. Researchers have documented that patient participation in the health care experience can lead to better outcomes, fewer disease-related limitations, more efficient use of resources, and improved patient satisfaction.[1] Moreover, active involvement by patients in their own care is vital because patient knowledge, self-observation, and feedback to the providers are routinely needed for sound medical decision making. The effect of active patient and family involvement on reducing medical errors is still under investigation; however, anecdotal results are promising.[2]

Provision of safe health care services is an objective for every health care provider. It is in everyone's best interests to prevent untoward side effects, treatment-related injuries, communication failures, and technical mishaps. Active involvement of patients in the health care experience provides another safety check in health care processes. By paying attention to the care being provided to them, patients can alert caregivers to potential errors so that corrective actions can be initiated before any harm occurs. For purposes of patient safety improvement, it is incumbent on all providers to embrace patients and family members as active participants on the health care team.

How Patients Can Help

Patients can help health care professionals do their jobs safely and protect themselves from harmful mistakes by taking the following actions:

- Talking with caregivers—telling about their history, problems they have had in the past, medications they have been taking, what is confusing to them, and what concerns they may have

- Reminding caregivers to confirm their identity before administering any medication or treatment and by speaking up if it appears the caregiver has them confused with someone else

- Confirming that caregivers know what the doctor has ordered for them and that the caregivers have all the information needed in order to provide safe care

- Telling caregivers about their allergies to any medications or food and reminding everyone to communicate information about their allergies to food and medications to other members of the health care team

- Informing caregivers if they have been taking any medicinal herbal products or over-the-counter medications, which can help prevent unnecessary drug-to-drug or drug-to-food interactions and adverse drug reactions

- Giving caregivers any medications they have brought to the hospital from home so that potential interactions with other medications or other injuries can be prevented

- Asking caregivers to explain the medications that are being offered to verify if it is the right medication for them; if not, questioning the caregiver's decision to administer the medication

- Asking questions about their care plan so that they fully understand what they need to do and how they should do it, including how to change dressings and the frequency and dosage of their medications
- Telling their surgeon or anesthesia professional about all of their health conditions, any allergic reactions, and the medications they take
- Asking hospital staff members if they have reviewed the history and physical report that was provided by their primary doctor or surgeon
- Asking questions about the risks involved with anesthesia and/or medications they will receive during a surgery or a procedure
- Reminding caregivers to verify the site of the procedure so that everyone knows where the procedure will be performed and asking the surgeon to mark the site so there is no confusion in the operating room or procedure area
- Asking caregivers to explain why a test or treatment may be needed and how it might help them in order to identify an incorrect order for a test or a test that is meant for another patient
- Asking about test results, what they mean, and how they will be addressed
- Asking about the equipment used in their care to understand what different sounds or noises mean so they can notify caregivers if it appears there may be a potential problem[3]

Active patient involvement is the right thing to do, but this goal can be difficult to achieve. As the primary beneficiaries of health care services (and the recipients of any medical errors), patients, it would seem, have the most to gain from improvements in safety. Yet practitioners may find it challenging to engage patients and family members in error prevention activities; some people appear satisfied to remain uninvolved and uninformed. There are also barriers that originate from health care professionals themselves. Patriarchal attitudes, ineffective communication skills, and perceived lack of time are just some of the impediments to helping patients become active participants in their own care. The common barriers on both sides of the patient-practitioner partnership are discussed in this chapter, along with strategies for reducing these obstacles.

The Empowered Patient

Improving the safety of health care services may depend in part on the patient's active involvement; some people, however, may not wish to be involved. Patients may be unaccustomed to active participation in health services delivery and consequently don't expect their caregivers to encourage them to do otherwise. Other patients are more demanding and critical of the care they receive. These people are offended when they are not treated as equal members of the health care team. Most patients are somewhere between these two extremes. The challenge for health care professionals is to understand how best to recognize and respond to the desires of the individual patient.

Factors Affecting Caregiver-Patient Partnerships

Put yourself in the place of a newly hospitalized patient. You feel miserable and frightened. The nurse asks your family to wash their hands each time they visit and also mentions that you should remind nurses to do the same thing in case they forget. Now, in addition to feeling miserable and frightened, you're confused. You may find yourself wondering, "Shouldn't my nurses always remember to wash their hands before touching me? I wonder what else they might forget to do?"

Inviting patients to be involved in safety reveals to them the risk of errors. Some patients will choose to shoulder responsibility for safer health care delivery, whereas others will be content to sit back and rely on health care professionals to do it right every time. A number of factors contribute to patients' willingness and ability to share safety improvement responsibilities.

Preoccupation with Other Issues

Patients may be wrestling with internal or external constraints that inhibit effective communication with practitioners. Patients may be worrying about family or employment issues or coping with a new diagnosis. They may be anxious about financial difficulties or may have unresolved personal matters. A patient who doesn't respond positively to suggestions for more active participation in the health care experience may very well be interested in participating but needs time to deal with personal issues first.

Fear

Some patients may not voice concerns about safety for fear of offending health care providers. In the past, caregivers may have rebuked the patient when he or she spoke up about unsafe situations or questioned health care practices. Health care professionals often tell patients not to worry and to put more trust in their providers. This can create a situation in which patients think their concerns won't be listened to or it won't do any good to express them. Some patients are fearful that raising questions might actually cause an error to occur or think their questions are not legitimate. Especially in situations where patients feel vulnerable, they don't want to be viewed by caregivers as being too demanding.

Denial

Although there has been considerable media attention on medical errors, patients often believe that an error won't happen to them. They have an almost blind faith in the ability of health care professionals to not make mistakes. Patients frequently don't appreciate that mistakes are often caused by breakdowns in the process of care, something that competent professionals can't always control. And even competent practitioners are fallible.

Indifference

Some patients resent being asked to participate in protecting themselves from mistakes that might be made during the delivery of health services. It's not uncommon to hear a patient say, "It is their job to take care of me; that's what they are getting paid for!" The traditional paternalistic attitude of health care professionals has contributed in no small way to this attitude.[4] All too often patients were—and are—expected to be passive and dependent rather than active coproducers of health care services.

Age and Condition

Some studies of patient participation in health care decision making suggest that older, sicker patients are more likely than others to be passive.[5] Unfortunately, these are the patients who stand to benefit the most from error prevention strategies because their care is usually complex and likely to involve multiple caregivers and sites of care. Older patients are typically not accustomed to being active health care participants and become anxious when practitioners encourage them to speak up. Younger patients tend to be more assertive; however, this attitude can change to passivity if the patient is faced with a life-threatening disease.

Education and Literacy

It is estimated that up to 90 million patients in the United States have some type of health illiteracy that negatively impacts their understanding of health care information. One study, for example, indicates that up to 40 percent of the respondents were unable to fully understand the information and warnings contained on a common prescription bottle.[6] Even people who can sign their names may lack the skills needed to assimilate verbal or written instructions communicated by caregivers. Patients with low literacy often feel embarrassed and therefore may not ask questions or reveal that they don't understand.

Language

English is not the primary language for many patients. Interpreters may be present for the diagnostic or treatment interactions with clinicians, but these are not always the ideal times for communicating information about safety. Written materials used to educate patients about their role in maintaining a safe environment can be confusing or misleading if translated literally into other languages.

Culture

Patients come from a wide variety of ethnic groups with diverse religious, social, and cultural beliefs. In some societies, it would be considered bad manners for the physician or nurse to ask the patient or family members to assist in preventing mistakes, so merely asking a patient to express safety concerns may not yield a satisfactory response. In many cultures, patients and family members accept the physician's decision or the nurse's direction without question. Patients may not be accustomed to making choices about their own health needs and would never think to point out a mistake that has been made. Stressful situations, such as a serious illness, can lead to even greater patient-practitioner communication difficulties.

Strengthening Patient Involvement

Questions that must be asked include, Do consumers want to be involved in the patient safety movement? To what extent is such an agenda paternalistic (i.e., guardians looking after the best interests of the consumers), and to what extent is it truly consumer driven? Past studies of patients' interest in shared health care decision making may provide a clue. There is compelling evidence to suggest that patient involvement in health care decisions has a positive effect on patient satisfaction, compliance with treatment recommendations, and outcomes.[7] For this reason, models of patient care that emphasize the patient's active involvement are being promoted. Researchers have discovered that some patients want to play no role in the decision process, and yet others want to take full control in the therapy selection.[8] Most studies suggest that only a minority of patients wish to assume the role of primary decision maker.

It is quite likely the same variation will be found when consumers are asked about being involved in the prevention of medical errors. Some people will express the belief that health care
providers should have sufficient knowledge and skills to prevent
mistakes, and health care processes should be designed more
safely. These people expect providers to function as the sole
guardians of safety. Other consumers will accept information
about their role in preventing medical errors but may not act on
the information unless providers are supportive. For these people, health care professionals must function in the role of friend
or teacher to encourage their involvement. For action to occur,
both the consumer and provider must believe that the patient's
active participation can have a positive impact on safety.

A third group of consumers deliberately seek out information on medical error prevention. These consumers may have
personally experienced a medical mishap and wish to deter
future problems, or they may be fearful of a mistake because of
media reports or discussions with friends or relatives.[9] Medical-
error prevention information may be obtained directly from
providers or other sources (e.g., consumer groups, medical professional associations, Internet health sites, support groups).
Even though these patients may have a limited understanding
of clinical care and associated processes, they may try to over-
see all aspects of health care safety. Some providers view this
group of consumers as "meddlers," which unfortunately can
widen the patient-practitioner communication gap. Caregivers
have a responsibility to assist proactive consumers in accessing,
understanding, and applying the information they need to be
more effective partners with the health care team.

One would presume that all consumers would embrace any
opportunity to prevent health services errors that might cause
personal harm. However, a recent study suggests otherwise.
In a 2005 survey of patients discharged from hospitals in the
Midwest, many reportedly asked questions about their care
(85 percent) and a medication's purpose (75 percent), but far
fewer confirmed they were the correct patient (38 percent),

helped mark their incision site (17 percent), or asked about hand washing (5 percent).[10] While the study authors found that patients were generally agreeable to partnering with caregivers, participation varied according to their level of comfort in taking different actions. Educational interventions to increase patients' comfort with error prevention strategies may be necessary to help patients become more engaged.

Patients cannot participate in safety improvement activities unless they have the right types of information, given in ways optimal for their own level of understanding. There is a compelling need for education and other interventions to communicate with consumers about how to improve the safety of their health care experience. True patient participation in safety requires that health care professionals have an awareness of patient expectations and perceived needs and the extent to which these needs are being adequately addressed.

Practice Implications

What does such awareness mean to health care professionals? For one thing, it doesn't mean that practitioners should give up trying to involve patients and their families in the patient safety movement. That would be irresponsible. Understanding the barriers to effective patient-practitioner partnerships is the first step toward designing better ways of encouraging and educating patients, especially those prone to passivity, to become active members of the health care team. The following strategies have proved successful.

Use Your Position

The status of health care professionals in the eyes of patients can be a benefit. Most patients, respectful of their physicians, nurses, and other caregivers, will respond well to an invitation to help out. By saying something like, "I will do my job better if you read this material or follow these suggestions," the clinician is inviting the patient to help make his or her job easier.

This approach encourages patients (and family members) to be involved with the practitioner in delivering safe care.

During the delivery of care, practitioners should serve as models for safe behaviors and point out what is being done for safety purposes. When the doctor states, "I'm checking your allergies before I prescribe this medication," the patient can see that even competent practitioners need reminders on occasion to prevent slipups. Patients will also realize the importance of sharing information about their allergies; otherwise, caregivers won't be able to do their job as effectively.

Facilitating patient participation in error reduction activities requires a time commitment from caregivers. The most anxiety-producing aspect of the patient-practitioner relationship is lack of time. If the caregiver doesn't allow sufficient time to discuss various strategies for reducing mistakes, the patient may be left with the nagging fear that safety is not a high priority for the provider. The basic problem is the time that effective communication requires. The rapid pace of health care, especially in acute care settings, can impede communication. Concern for other patients and the tasks that need to be completed can cause health care professionals to become distracted and to listen with only partial attention. Fatigue, stress, and anxiety that often stem from poor communication with other care providers; cumbersome information systems; and confusing protocols and procedures create barriers to spending time listening to patients and exploring their questions and concerns.[11] All of these pressures make health care professionals poor communication role models for patients.

How practitioners interact with patients can have a dramatic effect on whether patients are comfortable speaking up. Patients may be reluctant to raise issues or talk about concerns if they sense that the caregiver is uncomfortable or doesn't have time to engage in the discussion. This happens when health care professionals use "blocking behaviors" that discourage continued discussion.[12] Examples of blocking behaviors are listed in figure 4-1.

Figure 4-1.   Blocking Behaviors that Inhibit Practitioner-Patient Communication

- Defend an action we have taken, and block patients from continuing to express their concern.

- Interrupt and finish sentences of patients, cutting them off before they are able to express their concern in their own words.

- Talk more than patients do—making it difficult for them to squeeze their perspective into the conversation.

- Deliberately change the subject because we are uncomfortable. This shuts down everyone, except the most persistent patient, from being able to express concerns.

- Fail to clarify patients' concerns and run the risk of misunderstanding what they have said and taking an inappropriate course of action.

- Offer premature or inappropriate reasons or answers. We may be acting on too little information and misadvise patients. In these situations, patients may feel their concerns are being invalidated.

- Cite policy as the reason for an action. This communicates to patients that only hospital policy matters, not their needs or feelings.

- Overtly avoid an issue. This communicates a lack of interest in the patients' concerns and often shuts down dialogue with patients on other issues. This is a definite disincentive for patients to speak up again.

- Minimize patients' concern. Patients may lose face or feel they have overreacted or were just plain silly for speaking up at all.

- Disregard patients' concern with condescending comments such as, "We have got it handled." This conveys disrespect for patients' feelings and concerns.

- Make promises to do things we don't or can't follow through on. This jeopardizes patients' confidence and trust in everyone on the health care team.

- Put down the organization. This causes a loss of patients' trust in our ability to care for them safely. It compromises any respect we have been able to build with patients.

Patients learn a great deal about how to communicate with health care professionals by watching how practitioners interact with them. When clinicians model positive communication traits, those same traits can be cultivated in patients. Patients won't respond to an invitation to become an active health care participant simply because the practitioner tells them to. Patients want and deserve explanations about safety. When caregivers don't take sufficient time to explain, patients may begin to doubt the providers' commitment to keeping them safe.

Relinquish Paternalism

In ancient times, medicine was based on magic and religion. The Greco-Roman god of medicine, Aesculopius, was worshipped in hundreds of temples throughout Greece. The sick gathered at these temples for a healing ritual known as "incubation" or "temple sleep." While in a dream state, the sick were visited by Aesculopius or one of his priests who gave advice. According to ancient writings, many patients, on awakening, were cured of their ailments.

The science of medicine has changed considerably since ancient Greek and Roman times, although for centuries patients continued to be denied credibility or authority over their treatment, presumably because they were seen as "too sick" to be listened to. Attempts to guide patient decisions often tended toward paternalism rather than genuine empowerment. It wasn't until the last half of the twentieth century that consumers in some countries, including the United States, started to demand a more active and personal role in the health care experience.[13]

Broad societal changes have shifted the demands, expectations, and attitudes of health care consumers. Old-style paternalism, for all its achievements, is now a barrier to patient safety. Patients want caregivers who will be counselors and interpreters, not just guardians of knowledge.[14] Once health care professionals relinquish paternalistic attitudes, they are forced to develop and enhance their repertoire of communication skills: listening to patients, answering questions, helping patients make decisions, directing patients to appropriate resource materials, and being fellow learners.

Health care professionals often don't appreciate how patients can help prevent errors. The author informally polled physicians, nurses, and other health care professionals at five different hospitals to ascertain their views on patient involvement in the safety movement. She discovered that many practitioners thought patients and their families don't have the knowledge or ability to contribute to their own safety because laypersons are unable to fully comprehend the technical aspects of health care. Some hospital nurses expressed concerns that constant questions or reminders voiced by patients will interfere with nurses performing their work. Some nurses believed that asking patients to bring up safety concerns was more of a "customer service" than an intervention that would actually help reduce errors. These commonly held beliefs are being challenged by recent studies that demonstrate patients are able to identify adverse and near-miss events and can help prevent some of these events by questioning caregivers during service delivery.[15]

To effectively partner with consumers in the patient safety movement, health care professionals must become consultants, advisers, and confidantes. Fortunately, evidence in recent years is showing that many health service providers are increasingly recognizing the importance of patient participation, which involves listening to, and acting on, advice from patients. From the perspective of safety, health care consumers are in a unique position to identify problems and suggest solutions based on experiential knowledge.

Communicate from the Patient's Perspective

Effective communication is necessary if patients and their families are to become involved in preventing medical mishaps. Communication breakdowns can be caused by language differences and verbal misunderstandings as well as by cultural differences. Below is an example of a miscommunication incident reported by a hospital to the Pennsylvania Patient Safety Authority.

A patient with a dye allergy was ordered a CT scan with contrast. "No allergies" was noted on the admission orders. The allergy was noted on the medication administration record, but not on the patient care kardex. The nurse asked the patient if he had an allergy to "contrast," but the patient said "no" because he did not realize that the term meant IV dye. The patient was started on the contrast infusion and only later reported the allergy.[16]

Language differences may be easy to compensate for, but it is equally important—and perhaps more difficult—to overcome cultural barriers. A little knowledge, a lot of alertness, and the willingness to work within another person's cultural norms can go far toward creating better patient-practitioner partnerships.

All consumer materials related to patient safety should be available in the person's native language. This may seem an obvious suggestion for the non–English-speaking patient, but often health care professionals fail to recognize that people who can speak English may not be able to read English or may prefer reading in their own language. If English is a patient's second language, it is important to determine the patient's English proficiency and offer bilingual patient safety materials or interpreters. Many of the patient safety consumer education materials developed by the Agency for Healthcare Research and Quality are available in English and Spanish.[17] Organizations such as the University of Washington and Harborview Medical Center in Seattle have developed multilingual patient education materials.[18]

The value of practitioner sensitivity to cultural barriers cannot be underestimated. An important factor as it relates to patient safety is that 75 percent of cultures around the world are group oriented.[19] One of the many manifestations of this cultural value is the extreme importance of the extended family. Family members want to be involved in the patient's care and, if educated about safety along with the patient, can greatly increase the likelihood that the information will be retained and practiced. There are numerous other issues to consider when caring for patients from other ethnic groups; however, the topic is well beyond the scope of this chapter. A number of resources to assist health care professionals in understanding how to interact with patients from various cultures are listed in figure 4-2.

Figure 4-2. Cultural Diversity Resources for Health Care Professionals

Carolyn D'Avanzo and Elaine Geissler. *Pocket Guide to Cultural Assessment,* 3rd ed. (St. Louis: Mosby, 2002).

Center for Cross-Cultural Health, sponsored by the University of Minnesota: http://www.crosshealth.com.

Culture Clues™ tip sheets for clinicians to increase awareness about concepts and preferences of patients from the diverse cultures served by University of Washington Medical Center, Seattle: http://depts. washington.edu/pfes/cultureclues.html.

EthnoMed information Web site, sponsored by Harborview Medical Center, Seattle: http://www.ethnomed.org.

Geri-Ann Galanti. *Caring for Patients from Different Cultures,* 3rd ed. (Philadelphia: University of Pennsylvania Press, 2003).

Improving Cultural Competency in Children's Health Care (Cambridge, MA: National Initiative for Children's Healthcare Quality, 2005): http://www.nichq.org.

Leo S. Morales, Juan Antonio Puyol, and Ron D. Hays. *Improving Patient Satisfaction Surveys to Assess Cultural Competence in Health Care* (Oakland, CA: California HealthCare Foundation, 2003): www. chcf.org/documents/consumer/PatientSurveysCulturalCompetence.pdf.

Network for Multicultural Health, Center for Health Professions, University of California, San Francisco: http://futurehealth.ucsf.edu/ TheNetwork.

Rachael E. Spector. *Cultural Diversity in Health and Illness,* 6th ed. (Upper Saddle River, NJ: Prentice Hall, 2003).

Rani Srivastava. *The Healthcare Professional's Guide to Clinical Cultural Competence* (Philadelphia: W. B. Saunders Co., 2006).

Literacy also affects patient-practitioner communication. Patients with low literacy can misunderstand verbal or written communications. Recognizing this as problematic, the U.S. Department of Health and Human Services mandated in its *Healthy People 2010* report that all health care communications designed for patients be scrutinized for an appropriate reading comprehension level. In this case, *appropriate* is defined as the reading comprehension level congruent with the reading level of the majority of patients. Too often, printed materials baffle patients because authors don't take into account the users' literacy level, reading skills, thinking style, or short-term memory.

All written patient safety education materials should be tested for readability. One way to test for readability is to use readability software to make sure the target population can read the booklets. But writing at a lower-grade level may not be more understandable if some of the other issues, such as type size and line length, aren't addressed. An even better idea is to ask patients and family members to help evaluate and rewrite the materials. See chapter 5 for an extensive discussion of how health literacy affects patient and family collaboration efforts and what can be done to minimize the impact.

Keep Patients Informed

Patients are frequently told to speak up when they have a concern. Yet how many patients know the difference between what should be happening and what is actually happening? For patients to serve as effective system safeguards, it is vital for them to know more about the health care process. For example, clinic patients should be told when to expect to hear back from their physician (or their designee) about diagnostic test results.

The patient should be told to initiate contact with the physician if no communication has been received within a specified period. Patients may believe that "no news is good news" when, in fact, test results may have never been delivered to the physician. The patient-initiated contact with the physician might be the last line of defense in making sure test results get to the right place.

Some hospitals have created informational brochures or patient education tools that explain what will happen during hospitalization. An example of a patient version of a clinical path is shown in figure 4-3. The clinical pathway describes in layperson terms what is most likely to happen during a patient's hospital stay for heart failure. Caregivers use this document as a teaching tool for the patient as well as family members. The "Your Responsibility" section on the pathway suggests ways in which the patient can partner with caregivers to improve outcomes and reduce unintended adverse events. Armed with a better understanding of what is likely to happen, patients can now become active participants. It is easier for patients or family members to speak up when something doesn't seem quite right if they know what to expect and have been encouraged to partner with caregivers. Providing process transparency, where it makes sense, allows patients to be more involved in error prevention.

Widespread support is given to the idea that the partnership between practitioners and patients should be improved and strengthened. Furnishing better and timely information to patients is an essential element of health service safety. A revolutionary way of keeping patients informed about the health care experience has begun in the United Kingdom. This initiative involves providing patients with copies of clinician-to-clinician letters and is intended as a way to increase patients' involvement in their care and treatment and keep them up to date on all matters related to their health.

A common complaint by patients is that doctors and nurses talk about them as if they weren't there. So why should clinicians correspond with one another about patients without including the patients in the information loop? Supporters of the United Kingdom initiative suggest that copying letters to patients involves them more personally in their care.[20] Commenting in support of the project, Harry Cayton, director of

Figure 4-3. Heart Failure Patient Pathway, Boston Medical Center

BOSTON MEDICAL CENTER

HEART FAILURE
PATIENT PATHWAY

ADMISSION	DURING YOUR STAY	DISCHARGE	GENERAL GOALS

• You will begin to meet the staff who will care for you
  Doctors A group will be in charge of your care led by your Attending Physician
  Nurses Create, explain, deliver and monitor your plan of care
  Physical Therapists Monitor and progress your activity
  Dietician Reviews necessary dietary changes
  Case Coordinator Plans for and arranges services you might need after the hospital
• You will be examined by a doctor and have necessary blood tests and other tests to examine your heart
• You may have an intravenous line (IV) inserted in your arm to give medications and if needed you may receive oxygen to help your breathing
• Your healthcare team will teach you
  ◇ About your surroundings
  ◇ The importance of reporting any symptoms
	• You will be examined by your doctor
	• Your doctor will discuss all test results with you
	• You will be weighed
	• What you drink and what you put out in urine will be monitored by your nurse
	• You may have an EKG, Echocardiogram and/or other tests to examine your heart's function
	• IV medications will be changed to medications in a pill form as you get better
	• You may be seen by the Physical Therapist to increase your strength
	• Your healthcare team will teach you
	  ◇ Importance of reporting symptoms or changes in your condition
	  ◇ Energy conservation skills
	  ◇ How to maintain a daily weight and watch fluid/salt intake
	  ◇ About your medications and when you should take them
	  ◇ About low salt diet
	  ◇ Counsel you about not smoking if you are a smoker
		• You will be examined by your doctor
		• Your doctor will answer any final questions you might have, discuss any changes to medications you will take at home and okay your discharge from the hospital
		• You may have blood work and an EKG
		• You will be given activity guidance by your Physical Therapist
		• You will be given a follow up appointment with your Primary Care Physician and Cardiologist
		• Your healthcare team will teach you
		  ◇ About your home medications and when you should take them
		  ◇ Remind you to take no other medications than the ones we have prescribed
		  ◇ About daily weight monitoring
		  ◇ What to do if symptoms worsen
		  ◇ When to call
		  ◇ **Plan for your ride to pick you up between 10am - 12pm**
			• We want you to be able to manage your heart failure and to enjoy your life without heart symptoms
			• Your GOALS
			  ◇ Take an active role in your heart failure management
			  ◇ Have a plan with your healthcare team for managing any symptoms
			
			As you leave the hospital, you should be able to answer "YES" to following statements If not, please be sure to review any areas with you
			
			1 ☐ I have been given heart failure information packet
			2 ☐ I have a scale to weigh myself at home
			3 ☐ I understand what heart failure is
			4 ☐ I know what to do if symptoms worsen
			5 ☐ I know when I should take my medications
			6 ☐ I understand what my medications are for an what side effects to watch out for
			7 ☐ I have a way to get my prescriptions today
			8 ☐ I understand how to weigh myself daily and to contact my physician for a weight gain of 2 - 3 lbs over 1 - 2 days
			9 ☐ I understand my home activity program
			10 ☐ I understand a low salt diet
			11 ☐ I know the resources to help me quit smoking if I smoke
			12 ☐ I feel confident of my abilities to care for myself at home
			13 ☐ I know when and with whom my follow up appointments are
			14 ☐ I have been given personalized script to BMC's cardiovascular website

Your Responsibility	**Your Responsibility**	**Your Responsibility**	
• Inform your nurse immediately if ANY chest discomfort, difficulty breathing, dizziness or irregular heartbeat occur • To share any concerns you may have • To ask any questions you may have	• Inform your nurse immediately if ANY chest discomfort, difficulty breathing, dizziness or irregular heartbeat occur • To discuss any questions you have • Learn to monitor daily weights and keep daily diary of your weight • To recognize sources of salt in your diet • **Day prior to discharge, please let family know you will be discharged between 10am -12pm.**	• To discuss any questions you may have • To create a discharge medication schedule that fits your life style • To keep follow up appointments • To take an active role as you go home in management of your heart failure	

TO BE GIVEN TO PATIENT / FAMILY

DT99910089HEARTFALPWKIT

Rev 4/04 BMB 101000

Source: Boston Medical Center, Boston, Massachusetts, 2004. Reprinted with permission.

Patient Experience and Public Involvement, United Kingdom Department of Health, noted that the new relationship between health professionals and service users requires openness, mutual respect, sharing of expertise, and joint decision making. Copying physicians' letters to patients is one small step on the way to rebalancing the patient-practitioner relationship—but a symbolic and important one.[21] The response of health care consumers in the United Kingdom has been very positive. A patient from one of the pilot sites for copying letters to patients said, "It lets you know what the hospital knows. There should be no secrets, no constraints—generally, I thought it was brilliant. In the past you didn't get to know anything. You walked into the hospital grounds not knowing anything."[22]

There are, of course, practical matters to be considered in copying letters to patients: patient consent, security, confidentiality, and the ability of practitioners to be technically precise while reasonably comprehensible. These issues are not insurmountable, but it would be unfortunate if health care professionals were unwilling to tackle the issues merely because copying letters to patients might require a change in usual health service work practices.

Education and knowledge are empowering forces for patients wishing to take an active role in the health care experience, and providers must support this role. Carl Carpenter, PhD, a member of the board at Regional Medical Center in Orangeburg, South Carolina, feels strongly that hospitals must become more involved in creating partnerships with patients. "Physicians, nurses, and other health care providers have to become better 'facilitators of learning' for patients, and we've got to support that transition. Trustees should be asking: 'What can our hospital do to help strengthen patient-caregiver collaboration?'"[23]

Be Open and Honest

Health care professionals can work in partnership with patients in a number of ways. By offering explanations about procedures that will be performed, medications that will be administered, or other activities that will be conducted, practitioners are giving patients an opportunity to act as a safeguard in the process. Patient-practitioner dialogue cannot be just one sided. There should be a back-and-forth exchange of information. And this means that it is hoped patients will communicate their safety concerns to practitioners. To maintain open dialogue with patients, caregivers must be adequately prepared to respond when one of those patients says, "I think you may have made a mistake." Such statements can cause clinicians to become defensive and seek ways of disengaging or discrediting the discussion. Doctors Chassin and Becher described this phenomenon in an article about the case of a patient who was mistakenly taken for another patient's invasive electrophysiology procedure. Despite the patient's repeated objections, the practitioners discounted what the patient was saying. The physicians and nurses believed the patient lacked information about the planned procedure.[24]

Health care activities are often very confusing to patients, so it's reasonable that patients or family members may perceive a situation inaccurately. In addition, how caregivers respond to inquiries influences patients' willingness to voice other concerns. If a mistake has not been made, caregivers should explain the situation because it's important to acknowledge the validity of patients' concerns and apologize for any confusion or lack of communication that may have occurred. Caregivers should thank patients and families for paying attention and congratulate them for asking questions. Encourage patients to speak up again by explaining that mistakes sometimes do occur and it is helpful for them to be vigilant.

If a patient's inquiry results in the realization that a mistake has been made, caregivers must take responsibility, apologize, and act to mitigate or correct the error or concern. Do not be defensive when this situation occurs. The patient-practitioner dialogue should go something like this: "Thank you for telling me. I'm sorry this happened, and I understand why you are upset. This is what I am going to do about it. I will get back to you in a little while and make sure everything has been resolved."

Reducing errors is a major challenge for health care organizations. The practitioner's response to patients' questions, concerns, and feedback will directly influence how willing patients are to assist in preventing or intercepting errors.

Working Together for Safety

Studies suggest that consumer faith and confidence in the medical profession have been eroding in the United States as well as in many other Western nations. Growing consumer skepticism about the quality and safety of patient care will lead toward less deferential, more informed, and more demanding patients. If health care professionals want to enlist the help of patients in preventing medical mistakes, new patient-practitioner relationships must be formed.

It should be no surprise that *Marcus Welby, MD,* was one of the most popular doctor shows in American television history. During the 1970 television year, it ranked number one among all TV series.[25] The scripts, authored by writer-physician Michael Halberstam, portrayed an idealized doctor-patient relationship characterized by Welby's incredibly solicitous and loyal bedside manner. Welby's demeanor undoubtedly influenced the public's image of the ideal practitioner. Some members of the medical profession even claimed that Welby was among the factors contributing to the rise of malpractice actions against physicians in the 1970s.[26]

To effectively engage health care consumers in safety improvement, it is not necessary for health care professionals to be just like Dr. Welby. However, patients and their families do expect to be reassured, supported, and provided with adequate explanations. Practitioners must reach out to the patient and the patient's family to involve them in issues of safety to the extent that the patient and family are capable or wish to be involved.

Greater understanding about the risks inherent in the health care system is fundamentally useful for patients. If patient education is to make a difference in the safety of health services, however, practitioners must understand and overcome barriers that can undermine the value of patient involvement. No one has more interest in health care safety than patients. Health care professionals must accept patients as partners, trust their expertise, and allow them to help transform health care into a safer system.

References

1. S. Greenfield, S. Kaplan, and J. E. Ware, "Expanding Patient Involvement: Effects on Patient Outcomes," *Annals of Internal Medicine* 102, no. 4 (1985): 520–28; D. M. Vickery, T. J. Golaszewski, E. C. Wright, and H. Kalmer, "The Effect of Self-Care Interventions on the Use of Medical Services within a Medicare Population," *Medical Care* 26, no. 6 (1988): 580–88; D. Brody and others, "Patient Perception of Involvement in Medical Care: Relationship to Illness Attitudes and Outcomes," *Journal of General Internal Medicine* 4, no. 6 (1989): 506–11; P. D. Mullen, "Compliance Becomes Concordance," *British Medical Journal* 314, no. 7082 (1997): 691.

2. S. A. Weigman and M. R. Cohen, "The Patient's Role in Preventing Medication Errors," in *Medication Errors,* M. Cohen, ed. (Washington, DC: American Pharmaceutical Association, 2002); E. J. Sobo, G. Billman, L. Lim, J. W. Murdock, E. Romero, D. Donoghue, W. Roberts, and P. S. Kurtin, "A Rapid Interview Protocol Supporting Patient-Centered Quality Improvement: Hearing the Parent's Voice in a Pediatric Care Unit," *Joint Commission Journal of Quality Improvement* 28, no. 9 (2002): 498–509.

3. M. H. Pelling, *Staying Safe: Your Role in the Healthcare Environment* (video) (Carrollton, TX: PRIMEDIA Healthcare, 2001).

4. C. Laine and F. Davidoff, "Patient-Centered Medicine: A Professional Evolution," *Journal of the American Medical Association* 275, no. 2 (1996): 152–56.

5. A. M. Stiggelbout and M. Gwendoline, "A Role of the Sick Patient: Patient Preferences Regarding Information and Participation in Clinical Decision-Making," *Canadian Medical Association Journal* 157, no. 4 (1997): 383–89.

6. J. Moisan, M. Gaudet, J. P. Grégoire, and R. Bouchard, "Noncompliance with Drug Treatment and Reading Difficulties with Regard to Prescription Labeling among Seniors," *Gerontology* 48, no. 1 (2002): 44–51.

7. C. M. Ruland, "Improving Patient Outcomes by Including Patient Preferences in Nursing Care," *Proceedings of the AMIA Symposium* (1998): 448–52; M. Heisler, R. R. Bouknight, R. A. Hayward, D. M. Smith, and E. A. Kerr, "The Relative Importance of Physician Communication, Participatory Decision Making, and Patient Understanding in Diabetes Self-Management," *Journal of General Internal Medicine* 17, no. 4 (2002): 243–52; S. H. Kaplan, S. Greenfield, and J. E. Ware, "Assessing the Effects of Physician-Patient Interactions on the Outcomes of Chronic Disease," *Medical Care* 27 (suppl) (1989): S100–S127.
8. R. B. Deber, N. Kratschmer, and J. Irvine, "What Role Do Patients Wish to Play in Treatment Decision Making?" *Archives of Internal Medicine* 156, no. 13 (1996): 1414–20; J. Benbassat, D. Pilpel, and M. Tidhar, "Patients' Preferences for Participation in Clinical Decision Making: A Review of Published Surveys," *Behavioral Medicine* 24, no. 2 (1998): 81–88; B. McKinstry, "Do Patients Wish to Be Involved in Decision Making in the Consultation? A Cross Sectional Survey with Video Vignettes," *British Medical Journal* 321, no. 10 (2000): 867–71.
9. *Update on Consumers' Views of Patient Safety and Quality Information* (Menlo Park, CA: Kaiser Family Foundation, 2006).
10. A. D. Waterman, T. H. Gallagher, J. Garbutt, B. M. Waterman, V. Fraser, and T. E. Burroughs, "Brief Report: Hospitalized Patients' Attitudes about and Participation in Error Prevention," *Journal of General Internal Medicine* 21, no. 4 (2006): 367–70.
11. E. B. Larson, "Measuring, Monitoring, and Reducing Medical Harm from a Systems Perspective: A Medical Director's Personal Reflections," *Academic Medicine* 77, no. 10 (2002): 993–1000.
12. C. Foster, *There's Something I Have to Tell You. How to Communicate Difficult News in Tough Situations* (New York: Harmony Books, 1997).
13. C. Laine and F. Davidoff, "Patient-Centered Medicine: A Professional Evolution," *Journal of the American Medical Association* 275, no. 2 (1996): 152–56.
14. D. G. Safran, "Defining the Future of Primary Care: What Can We Learn from Patients?" *Annals of Internal Medicine* 138, no. 3 (2003): 248–55; D. S. Main, C. Tressler, A. Staudenmaier, K. A. Nearing, J. M. Westfall, and M. Silverstein, "Patient Perspectives on the Doctor of the Future," *Family Medicine* 34, no. 4 (2002): 251–57.
15. S. N. Weingart, O. Pagovich, D. Z. Sands, J. M. Li, M. D. Aronson, R. B. Davis, D. W. Bates, and R. S. Phillips, "What Can Hospitalized Patients Tell Us about Adverse Events? Learning from Patient-Reported Incidents." *Journal of General Internal Medicine* 20, no. 9 (2005): 830–36; P. K. Greenhouse, B. Kuzminsky, S. C. Martin,

and T. Merryman, "Calling a Condition H(elp)," *American Journal of Nursing* 106, no. 11 (2006): 63–66.

16. Pennsylvania Patient Safety Authority, "When Patients Speak—Collaboration in Patient Safety," *Patient Safety Advisory* 2, no. 1 (2005): 1. [http://www.psa.state.pa.us/psa/lib/psa/advisories/v2n1march 2005/vol_2-1-march-05-article_a-patients_speak.pdf]. Accessed October 2007. Used with permission.

17. Materials are available for download on the Web site of the Agency for Healthcare Research and Quality [www.ahrq.gov].

18. University of Washington Health Sciences Library and Harborview Medical Center's Community House Calls Program, EthnoMed [http:www.ethnomed.org/]. Accessed October 2007.

19. D. Dysart-Gale, "Cultural Sensitivity Beyond Ethnicity: A Universal Precautions Model," *Internet Journal of Allied Health Sciences and Practice* 4, no. 2 (2006) [http://ijahsp.nova.edu/articles/vol4num1/dysart-gale.pdf]. Accessed October 2007.

20. C. Chantler and J. Johnson, "Patients Should Receive Copies of Letters and Summaries," *British Medical Journal* 325, no. 7360 (2002): 388–89.

21. Harry Cayton, director of Patient Experience and Public Involvement, United Kingdom Department of Health, London, "Copying Letters to Patients" (keynote speech), October 30, 2002 [http://www.dh.gov.uk/en/News/Speeches/Speecheslist/DH_4097895]. Accessed October 2007.

22. D. Jelley and T. van Zwanenberg, "Copying GP Referral Letters to Patients: Study of Patients' Views," *British Journal of General Practice* 50, no. 457 (2000): 657–58.

23. P. L. Spath, "Sharing the Knowledge," *Health Forum Journal* 46, no. 2 (2003): 16–19, 47.

24. M. R. Chassin and E. C. Becher, "The Wrong Patient," *Annals of Internal Medicine* 136, no. 11 (2002): 826–33.

25. "Marcus Welby, M.D.: U.S. Medical Drama," Museum of Broadcast Communications (Chicago) [http://www.museum.tv]. Accessed October 2007.

26. J. Turow, *Playing Doctor: Television, Storytelling, and Medical Power* (New York: Oxford University Press, 1989).

5

Integrating Health Literacy into Patient Safety Partnerships

*Cezanne Garcia and Cindy Brach**

Efforts to improve patient safety have rapidly expanded in the past decade. Initially, these initiatives were largely professionally driven, formulated and conducted by health professionals. However, growth of the patient- and family-centered care movement is reshaping the patient safety field. The confluence of patient safety and patient- and family-centered care has produced the realization that patients and family members have an important role in creating safe health care systems. Patients and family bring experience and wisdom to a partnership with health care professionals and organizations working to create an error-free care experience.

The patient and family role in patient safety is perhaps clearest in avoiding errors that stem from poor communication in the clinician-patient interaction. Patients and family members need to provide accurate medical histories and descriptions of symptoms, understand treatment choices, share in the decision making, and obtain knowledge and skills to safely manage their health conditions. Patients or family members lacking sufficient health literacy are less able to effectively partner with caregivers. Health care organizations

*As contributors to this book, we are grateful to the leaders in health care and literacy, including patient and family partners, who generously shared their experiences with us on their work to strengthen safety, health literacy, and patient- and family-centered care practices. We are likewise grateful to our families, who supported us through the preparation of this chapter and who enriched our understanding of health care and how it needs to change.

now appreciate that addressing health literacy is an essential component of patient safety.

The explicit connection between health literacy and patient safety was only made recently. The Institute of Medicine (IOM), in its landmark 2004 health literacy report, noted that inattention to cultural competence and health literacy can compromise patient safety.[1] The IOM also noted that patient inclusion in patient safety requires appreciation of the cultural nuances in people's understanding of safe care and the central role communication processes play. In 2006, the American Medical Association (AMA) Foundation sponsored the first health literacy and patient safety conference. Participants examined the link between limited health literacy and medication safety, considered how to measure effective communication practices, and explored the organizational changes necessary to promote a safer and shame-free environment. The following year saw the publication of the first two major reports on improving health literacy as a means to increasing patient safety: the AMA Foundation's *Reducing the Risk by Designing a Safer, Shame-Free Health Care Environment* and the Joint Commission's *What Did the Doctor Say? Improving Health Literacy to Protect Patient Safety*.[2] According to the Joint Commission, "Health literacy issues and ineffective communications place patients at greater risk of preventable adverse events."[3] This observation launches a series of recommendations for health care systems to incorporate health literacy strategies into the delivery of health care.

Health literacy strategies have tended to be clinician centered, with practitioners viewing patients' health literacy as a problem. Like traditional patient safety initiatives, the strategies have focused more on the one-way flow of information from clinicians to patients rather than on two-way information sharing and collaborative partnership. Although health literacy initiatives improve communication and make the health care system more navigable, they often put the onus of safeguarding patients squarely on the shoulders of professionals, rather than creating a strengths-based partnership model with patients and their families.

In this chapter we look at the intersection of patient safety and health literacy through the lens of patient and family partnering. First, we define and describe health literacy and examine what health literacy techniques have to offer the patient safety field. Then we explore how engaging patients and families as partners can bolster health literacy's contribution to creating a safe care experience. We describe promising approaches to sharing health information to improve patient safety and strengthening patients and families' ability to act on patient safety information. Finally we explore how patient- and family-centered partnerships and clear communication in patient safety improvement teams can transform the health care enterprise.

Health Literacy in the United States

Health literacy is defined by the U.S. Department of Health and Human Services as "the degree to which individuals have the capacity to obtain, process, and understand basic health information and services needed to make appropriate health decisions."[4] Health literacy, however, is not solely a characteristic of the individual.[5] Rather, it is the product of individuals' capacities *and* the demands that the health information places on individuals to decode, interpret, and assimilate health messages.[6] Furthermore, health literacy is not constant, but it is a dynamic state that may change with the situation.[7] For example, a patient's health literacy may plummet when he or she is presented with a cancer diagnosis.

Health literacy has to be differentiated from literacy. Literacy involves the ability to use print material. Health literacy is a much broader concept that encompasses both oral and written communication and the ability to act upon the communication. Health literacy can include specific health knowledge, familiarity with how the health care system works, as well as the ability to understand and use written and orally communicated health information.

Although it is widely agreed that health literacy is not limited to comprehending written materials in health care contexts, health literacy research and measurement tools have tended to default to literacy-based notions. The only national health literacy data, from the 2003 National Assessment of Adult Literacy (NAAL), measure only the ability to understand and use health-related printed information.[8] Even this limited set of data is revealing. The NAAL indicates that most Americans have difficulty understanding and acting upon printed health information.

- Only 12 percent of adults have *proficient* health literacy. In other words, nearly nine out of every ten adults may lack the skills needed to manage their health and prevent disease.
- Fourteen percent of adults (30 million people) have *below basic* health literacy—meaning that they are either nonliterate in English or can perform no more than the most simple and concrete health literacy skills, such as circling the date of a medical appointment on an appointment slip.
- An additional 22 percent (47 million people) have *basic* health literacy—indicating that they can perform only simple health literacy activities, such as locating one piece of information in a short document.

Some adults are more likely to have limited health literacy, including the poor; individuals who have limited English proficiency; individuals in poorer health; adults age 65 and older; and American Indian/Alaskan Native, black, and Hispanic adults.

The effects of limited literacy, as documented in the Agency for Healthcare Research and Quality (AHRQ) evidence report *Literacy and Health Outcomes,* carry numerous and serious consequences:[9]

- Adults with limited literacy are less likely to use preventive health services, such as mammograms, Pap smears, flu and pneumonia vaccines, and regular well-child visits for their children.

- Many disease management tools and approaches to develop self-management goals have not successfully served adults with limited literacy. For example, limited literacy adults with asthma are less likely to know how to use an inhaler, and limited literacy adults with diabetes are less likely to achieve hemoglobin A1c goals.

- Tools designed to teach understanding of medical concepts and strengthen shared decision making may not succeed if not designed for adults with varying health literacy skills. For example, a shared decision-making CD-ROM program for prostate cancer patients did not meet the needs of limited literacy patients.

Health literacy's prominence as a national health care priority has grown in recent years. Figure 5-1 traces health literacy's ascendancy over the past dozen years, highlighting the involvement of a growing number of federal and professional organizations. The following sections show how health literacy efforts have been or could be integrated with patient safety and how partnering with patients and their families helps improve these efforts.

Helping Patients and Families Understand Patient Safety Information

Many health literacy techniques have been developed to increase patients and families' understanding of oral communication and print materials and to make the health care system accessible to patients and families. Combining these techniques with patient- and family-centered approaches creates an environment in which constructive sharing of information can occur.

Figure 5-1.   Health Literacy's Ascendancy

- Plain Language movement (1995)
- *Healthy People 2010* goal: Increase Americans' health literacy (2000)
- Institute of Medicine's *Priority Areas for National Action*: Health literacy designated one of two cross-cutting priority areas (2001)
- American College of Physicians Foundation's Health Communication Initiative (2001)
- Establishment of the U.S. Department of Health and Human Services' Health Literacy Workgroup (2003)
- American Medical Association's *Health Literacy: Help Your Patients Understand CME Training* (2003)
- Institute of Medicine's *Health Literacy: A Prescription to End Confusion* (2004)
- Agency for Healthcare Research and Quality's *Literacy and Health Outcomes* (2004)
- National Center for Educational Statistics's *The Health Literacy of America's Adults: Results from the 2003 National Assessment of Adult Literacy* (2006)
- U.S. Surgeon General's Workshops on Improving Health Literacy (2006)
- American Medical Association Foundation's Health Literacy and Patient Safety Conference (2006)
- Joint Commission's *What Did the Doctor Say? Improving Health Literacy to Protect Patient Safety* (2007)
- American Medical Association Foundation's *Reducing the Risk by Designing a Safer, Shame-Free Health Care Environment* (2007)

Oral Communication

Patients' ability to understand and safely act upon health information is based on clear communication between patients and care providers. Health literacy principles suggest that clinicians should do the following:[10,11]

- Use plain, nonmedical language.
- Show or draw pictures and/or use three-dimensional models.
- Limit the amount of information provided.

- Repeat important information to enhance recall.
- Use "teach back" or "show me" techniques to confirm that patients and their families understand critical, need-to-know information.
- Provide easy-to-understand written materials to reinforce patient teaching.
  —Write the patient's name on these materials and check or circle key information, which encourages patient review after the care encounter.
  —Write down any unique information about which the patient inquires multiple times and that is not covered in the materials provided.
- Only provide written materials in conjunction with, and as reinforcement of, verbal instruction.
- Summarize the plan at the end of the care encounter.

These principles, however, are provider-centric. They focus on making what the clinician says understood by the patient. For example, the goal of the teach-back techniques described in figure 5-2 is to confirm that the patient understands the clinicians' instructions. If clinicians want to enhance understanding and create a patient- and family-centered approach to their care encounters, it is important that they also adopt the following behaviors:[12,13]

- Begin by asking patients and their families about their main concerns, and address these first.
- Ask the patients to prioritize their concerns; together, make a plan to address other concerns at subsequent visits or times during the hospitalization if too many issues are raised for one conversation.
- Explore the patients' conception of their illness—what caused it, what they fear about it, what results they would expect from treatment.
- Demonstrate understanding by empathic responses and familiarity with the patients' health and life history.

- Share options and encourage an active process of partnering with patients and their families to facilitate their decisions.

- Spend more time listening to patients and less time speaking.

- Encourage questions. Ask, "What questions do you have?" instead of, "Do you have any questions?"

Figure 5-2.   Teach-Back Techniques

Teach back is a method for checking patient understanding of health care information and instructions.[1] It is a prime tool in the health literacy arsenal and is also touted as an evidence-based patient safety practice.[2] Techniques include:

- Verify that the patient has understood instructions through use of the teach-back method. Ask the patient to recount what you have told him or her. You can use phrases such as:

  —"I want to make sure we have the same understanding. Tell me what you're going to do to keep your sugar under control."

  —"It's my job to explain things clearly. To make sure I did this, can you show me how you'd take this medicine at home?"

  —"Can you tell me, in your own words, the three things you said you would do between now and your next visit?"

- Review all information that is not fully understood using alternative approaches. Repeating exactly the same thing is unlikely to improve comprehension.

- Repeat the process until the patient indicates he or she has understood by correctly recounting the information. Make clear that the need to repeat is due to your failure to clearly convey the information rather than the "fault" of the patient. For example, you could say, "Let's talk about recording your weight because I think I have not explained it clearly."

- If you're concerned that teach-back will take too long, try it on your last patient before lunch or at the end of the day

[1] B. D. Weiss, *Health Literacy: A Manual for Clinicians* (Chicago: American Medical Association, 2003).

[2] Agency for Healthcare Research and Quality, *Making Health Care Safer: A Critical Analysis of Patient Safety Practices. Evidence Report/Technology Assessment*, No. 43 (Rockville, MD: Agency for Healthcare Research and Quality, 2001).

The combination of health literacy approaches with patient- and family-centered care practices makes it more likely that patients will understand health information and related safety practices and will act upon it.

Research shows that patients who leave doctors' offices with even one unanswered question reported the lowest level of improvement in their symptoms.[14] However, other studies show that patients who become more involved in their health care—including asking questions—are more likely to follow clinicians' instructions and report better results.[15,16]

Two major communication campaigns are currently under- way to encourage patients to take a more active role in the dialogue with clinicians. Ask Me 3, a health literacy campaign developed by the Partnership for Clear Health Communica- tion, encourages patients to pose the following three questions each time they talk with their health care provider: (1) What is my main problem? (2) What do I need to do? and (3) Why is it important for me to do this?[17] Questions are the Answer, an AHRQ patient safety campaign, encourages patients to ask questions as a way of preventing medical mistakes.[18] Both campaigns tested strategies and materials with consumers and involved the news media to directly reach consumers with their messages. Ask Me 3's Web site includes materials to help providers spread the message. Questions are the Answer's Web site features key resources to help patients become more involved with their health care, including the "Five Steps to Safer Health Care" fact sheet, a wallet-size question card, and an interactive "question builder" that encourages patients to develop a personalized list of questions to bring to each medi- cal appointment.

Written Materials

Well-designed written materials serve as effective remind- ers for patients and families of education and consultation communications with their clinicians.[19] Clearly written and well-designed materials have been demonstrated to improve comprehension of people at all literacy levels.[20] Furthermore, using illustrations that patients and families learn from, rather than those that merely look attractive, also increases comprehension, especially among those with low educational attainment.[21,22,23,24]

Health care organizations can adopt content and graphic standards as a means of incorporating durable best practices for enhancing health literacy.[25,26,27,28] (Figure 5-3 provides health literacy strategies for clear and easy-to-use written communications.) Adding an editor with health literacy expertise to the material development team can help the authors of written materials meet the needs of patients and families with varying health literacy levels.

Patients and families can play a powerful role in promoting information sharing, from instigating mutually beneficial dialogue to co-creating patient education materials. Patients and family members can serve as reviewers during the development phase to verify the suitability of messages. For example, at the University of Washington Medical Center, patients and family advisers are trained as material review advisers to evaluate drafted forms and educational materials. These advisers provide feedback to clinician authors to help:

- Clarify instructions and definitions of terms used in the medical safety field—such as *medical error, adverse event,* and *patient safety.*
- Address mismatches between instructions and content.
- Improve the layout logic and the sequence of ideas for knowledge and skill building.
- Strengthen readability.
- Distinguish between essential messages and peripheral information.
- Identify information that needs to be added to support the patient and family member's partner role in the care experience.

Figure 5-3.   Health Literacy Strategies for Clear and Easy-to-Use Written Communications

For all written materials:

- Use plain and clear language.
  - —Use short, simple, and familiar words (no jargon, acronyms, abbreviations)
  - —If you must use medical terms, define them the first time they are used
  - —Use short sentences that employ the active voice
  - —Write at sixth- to eighth-grade reading level
  - —Use culturally appropriate language

- Make content relevant.
  - —Limit the number of messages delivered
  - —Assume little or no background knowledge (especially about the human body and the healthcare system)
  - —Ensure that information is appropriately chunked
  - —Numbers and percentages are appropriate
    - –Provide only one number per point
    - –Calculations or inferences are not required
    - –Use easy-to-understand phrasing (e.g., one in ten instead of 10%)
    - –Use simple graphics that increase comprehension of text
    - –Remove extraneous information from displays: less is more
    - –When presenting quality and safety data, use "higher is better" terminology, which is more consistent with how individuals think
    - –Only use symbols in addition to or instead of numbers *if they have been audience tested*
  - —Use certified, professional, culturally competent interpreters and translators
  - —Graphic illustrations add value
    - –Clearly labeled with captions to explain graphics
    - –Must be directly applicable to text
    - –Must be simple and understandable
    - –Must be nondistracting and not busy
    - –Must be culturally appropriate

(Continued on next page)

Figure 5-3. (Continued)

- Format to enhance readability.
  —Use a lot of white space
  —Employ dark text on light background
  —Ensure ample space between lines (leading)
  —Use large type (at least 12-point) font, preferably serif
  —Justify left-hand margin only
  —Line length should be short (forty to fifty characters)
  —Break up text with bullets (avoid lengthy lists)
  —Use upper- and lowercase letters (no ALL CAPITAL WORDS)

- Conduct iterative testing.
  —Have materials reviewed by health literacy expert editors
  —Test with broad sample of intended patient/family members, which helps if you make sure reviewer group includes limited literacy and culturally diverse persons
    –Watch testers using it
    –Ask testers about their experience
    –Ask testers for editorial feedback
    –As appropriate, assess testers' comprehension
  —Test in all languages (if appropriate)

- Even with employing literacy-focused, easy-to-read materials, written materials must be used only as reinforcement to verbal interactive communications.

*Especially for Web sites:**

- Design for old hardware and software.
  —Site runs without requiring Flash, Shockwave, or other plug-ins
  —Loads relatively quickly, with no big graphics
  —Visuals clear on black and white monitor
  —Scales to smaller monitors
- Home page is simple.
- Information is prioritized.
  —Main point at top of page

---

*J. Eicher and P. Dullabh, *Accessible Health Information Technology (IT) for Populations with Limited Literacy: A Guide for Developers and Purchasers of Health IT* (Rockville, MD: Agency for Healthcare Research and Quality, 2007).

Creating a Shame-Free Environment

Communication begins with trust. The IOM's report *Preventing Medication Errors* reveals patients' expectations of the health care system.[29] These include being listened to and respected as a care partner, being told the truth, having care and information sharing coordinated with all members of the team, and partnering with staff who are able to provide both technically and emotionally supportive care. Creating a welcoming shame-free environment where patients and their families seek help when needed increases their confidence and comfort.[30,31] Following the guidelines below will help afford patients and their families respect and dignity at every point of contact.

- Encourage patients to bring family members or trusted friends to their appointments, and make accommodations for them in the room. Ask patients how they would like their family members or friends involved in their care.
- Greet patients warmly; first impressions count.
- Obtain interpreter services if the patient does not speak English.
- Have staff introduce themselves and provide explanations of their role in the care encounter.
- Ask patients and their families how they would like to be addressed (e.g., first name or surname, title).
- Give every patient the option to complete well-designed, easy-to-understand forms with the assistance of a staff member.
- Ask if there are cultural and/or spiritual practices that the patient would like to have accommodated to the extent possible in the care experience.
- Assure patients that many people have difficulty understanding health information.
- Distribute easy-to-read health brochures in appropriate languages.

- Offer alternatives to written health information (e.g., illustrations, audiotapes, videos, CD-ROMs) that can be viewed on-site or taken home.
- Provide clear directions to the office, laboratory, or referral location.
- Sit, if possible, when speaking to seated or bed-bound patients. Share diagnostic or treatment plan options with patients while they are dressed in their personal clothing rather than in a gown, or if hospitalized, with adequate bedding to accommodate their privacy and modesty needs.

The goal of creating a shame-free environment must be balanced with collecting important literacy information on patients. Clinicians are often encouraged to assess their patients' literacy, either by picking up on literacy red flags (see figure 5-4) or using a formal assessment tool, such as the Newest Vital Sign.[32,33] Many in the health literacy community, however, fear that subjecting patients to a literacy test will stigmatize them. Adults with limited literacy often keep it a secret, even from close friends and family, and avoid situations that risk exposure.[34,35] While some adults with limited literacy recount how they avoided doctors' offices because they did not want to have to reveal that they could not read or write, recent research suggests that most adults seen in clinical settings do not object to completing a literacy assessment.[36,37] More than 98 percent of patients, including a substantial proportion with limited literacy skills, were willing to undergo a literacy assessment in the course of routine clinical care, and performing such assessments did not decrease patient satisfaction.

Expecting clinicians to know each patient's literacy level and adapt communication styles accordingly may be taxing to already-strained practices. Perhaps adoption of universal health literacy precautions is more practical and consonant with creating a shame-free environment.[38,39] Universal health literacy precautions dictate that all patients be treated as if they

Figure 5-4.   Limited Literacy Red Flags

Behaviors

- Frequently missed appointments
- Noncompliance with medication regimens
- Lack of follow-through with laboratory tests, imaging tests, or referrals to consultants
- Patients say they are taking their medication, but lab tests or physiological parameters do not change in the expected fashion

Responses to Receiving Written Information

- Making excuses: "I forgot my glasses. I'll read this when I get home."
- Pretending to read
- Excessive clowning around, using humor

Responses to Request to Fill Out Forms

- Becoming angry and storming out
- Gripping pen tightly and taking a long time
- Incomplete or inaccurately completed forms

Responses to Questions about Medication Regimens

- Unable to name medications
- Unable to explain medication's purpose
- Unable to explain timing of medication administration
- Looking at pill instead of bottle label to identify medication

Source: Adapted from B. D. Weiss, *Help Patients Understand: A Manual for Clinicians* (Chicago: American Medical Association Foundation and American Medical Association, 2007), p. 17. Used with permission.

have limited health literacy because "you can't tell by looking." This does not imply that evidence of limited health literacy of particular patients should be ignored. It does mean, however, that clear communication techniques should be used with all patients, not only when limited health literacy is suspected. And if limited literacy skills are observed, documenting limited literacy in a patient's record could stimulate additional accommodations, such as a phone reminder of an appointment instead of just an appointment slip.

Clinician consensus on the need for universal health literacy precautions may be hard to achieve. Clinicians often overestimate the health literacy of their patients and may feel that changing their communication style is unnecessary.[40,41] A one-time literacy assessment of a sample of patients will give clinicians a sense of the patient population's literacy and could convince them that health literacy interventions are important to keep patients safe. For example, Community Health Partners in Livingston, Montana, has used the Newest Vital Sign to assess the literacy of all patients seen in a one-week period. According to Executive Director Laurie Francis, assessments are conducted periodically "to drive home the fact to all staff that a high percentage of our clients need various forms of communication to support their health/self-management goals, regardless of any evidence of low literacy and irrespective of highest grade in school attended."[42]

Helping Patients and Families Act on Patient Safety Information

A culture of safety supports and builds upon patient and family health literacy skills. Patients and families who work in partnership with health care providers to develop care plans and related goals are better able to act upon health information. While there is a health literacy dimension to many patient safety issues, three areas are particularly affected by health literacy—medication safety, informed consent, and self-management of chronic conditions.[43,44,45] Quality improvement trailblazers have initiated programs that focus on imparting skills to patients and their families to enable them to partner with their clinicians and take more control over their health and health care. Furthermore, health care providers are reaching out to community partners, particularly in the adult basic education community, to proactively improve patients' health literacy skills.

Medication Safety

The risk of patient harm due to medication errors has been well documented. Adverse events related to drugs are common in primary care, and many are preventable or ameliorable.[46] Research has shown that patients frequently do not understand the instructions on their prescription bottles and that communication between provider and patient regarding medication is insufficient.[47] A recent study showed that more patients made medication errors because of miscommunication between provider and patient (50 percent) than because they did not follow their medication regimen as they understood it (30 percent).[48] Care transitions, such as those at hospital admission and discharge, are particularly vulnerable to medication errors and adverse drug events.

Medication Review

Medication review, a comprehensive check on all medications—prescription, over the counter, herbal, and nutritional supplements—is a key process to reducing adverse drug interactions and improving patients' understanding of their medications and how to take them.

Increasingly, pharmacists are taking the lead on reviewing medications, a service now covered by Medicare and some Medicaid programs. The "brown bag" method of medication review consists of patients bringing in every medication and supplement they take routinely. Research in England has shown that patients perceived the following benefits from brown bag reviews: clinical problems resolved; better understanding of their medications, leading to increased confidence; and a sense of empowerment, resulting in their being more likely to be proactive in seeking information in the future.[49] Brown bag medication reviews appear to be a way of increasing patients' health literacy and building their skills to safely manage their conditions. The Ohio Patient Safety Institute created its Brown

Bag Toolkit, which can help pharmacists plan brown bag events and includes forms and checklists.[50]

Hospital Medication Reconciliation

The Joint Commission's Patient Safety Goal number 8 is to ensure that patients, their families, and clinicians have the most accurate and up-to-date medication list possible by means of a clinician-patient reconciliation process across the continuum of care.[51] Patients (or their designees) are given forms at every transition of care in which new medications are ordered or existing orders are rewritten. Responsible for contributing to the completion of a comprehensive and accurate medication list and identifying and clarifying discrepancies, patients and clinicians alike become alert to, and on guard against, potential medication errors.

Many health care facilities have collaborated with patients to design their strategies to meet this goal. For example, Children's Hospital and Regional Medical Center in Seattle found that parent advisers' involvement in its Rapid Process Improvement Workshop transformed implementation of medication reconciliation from regulatory requirement to "doing the right thing." By focusing on the family experience and listening to family input into the process design and forms, the team implemented a reliable process to collect a complete and accurate list of the patient's home medications, to compare the home medication list with any new medication orders for omissions and duplications, and to communicate the updated list to the family and next provider(s) of care.[52]

Some hospitals have also revised their discharge processes to help patients and families maintain postdischarge medication safety. For example, the Boston Medical Center developed and implemented a reengineered discharge (RED) intervention. RED consists of ten components, including a nurse "discharge advocate," a patient after-hospital care plan, and a follow-up call by a pharmacist several days after discharge. The after-hospital care plan contains reminders of medication allergies and a pill schedule that displays the names of all medicines the patient should take and the time of day, amount, and the method of taking. The plan was developed iteratively, using patient feedback to refine the packet and improve comprehension.

Informed Consent

"Ensuring that patients understand and consent to the healthcare interventions they receive is a basic component of patient safety."[53] So begins the National Quality Forum's (NQF) implementation report *Improving Patient Safety through Informed Consent for Patients with Limited Literacy.* Studies show that a substantial proportion of patients who have signed an informed consent form are unable to recall the major risks of surgery (18 to 45 percent) or do not know the exact nature of their operation (44 percent).[54,55,56,57] The consequences of providing care when true informed consent has not been obtained are exemplified by the case of Toni Cordell, a literacy advocate, who had a hysterectomy without her knowledge.[58] Stress and pain, which are known to cause patients' health literacy to drop, are often present when informed consent is obtained. Informed consent processes must therefore take into account that health literacy is a state, not a trait.

Informed consent forms can be improved by adopting the recommendations provided in figure 5-3 and the suggestions in the section above on written materials. Informed consent, however, is much more than a document; it is a process. Several efforts have been made to standardize and improve the process. For example, the NQF issued a specific recommendation in 2005 on how to implement one of its patient safety practices (Safe Practice Number 10): "Ask each patient or legal surrogate to recount what he or she has been told during the informed consent discussion." NQF issued a user's guide for implementing teach back and other key aspects of the informed consent process.

Several hospitals adopted teach back as part of their informed consent procedure. For example, the University of Virginia Health System responded to high rates of surgical delays and

rescheduling by asking patients at its Pre-Anesthesia Evaluation and Testing Center, "Can you tell me why you're here and
what you need to do before surgery?" to ensure that patients
understand preoperative instructions. The health system reported
avoiding adverse medication interactions and reducing the number of surgeries that had to be canceled or delayed due to patient
misunderstanding of instructions.[59] Successful implementation
of Safe Practice Number 10 benefits from standardizing the
process. San Francisco General Hospital not only uses teach
back to verify comprehension but has also instituted an informed
consent certification form. The certification form serves both as
a checklist and as documentation that all the appropriate information has been reviewed and a shared understanding reached
during the informed consent discussion.

Self-Management

An informed, active patient is in the center of the chronic care
model, a widely used framework for transforming the current
reactive health care system into one that uses planning, proven
strategies, and management to keep patients healthy.[60] Programs have emerged to improve patients' knowledge of their
conditions and their skills and confidence to improve self-care.
Increasingly, health information resource centers are taking
responsibility for helping patients and their families manage the
patient's health care.

The Chronic Disease Self-Management Program curriculum
developed by the Division of Family and Community Medicine
in the School of Medicine at Stanford University emphasizes
significant patient involvement in goal setting and a focus on
self-management in "real world" settings. Individuals/patients
living with chronic disease are recruited and trained as faculty
to facilitate the group self-management sessions. The program
concentrates on teaching problem-solving skills as a strategy
that strengthens safe care and focuses on medication adherence. The program showed that after one year, participants
had statistically significant improvements in a variety of health
outcomes and fewer emergency department visits.[61]

Blue Shield of California designed a patient-centered management strategy involving patients actively working with a care manager to develop shared goals and education strategies based on disease state, treatment options, pain management, and end-of-life decisions. This shared goal-planning strategy improved care coordination, effectively reduced overall costs by 26 percent, and resulted in high satisfaction scores among 92 percent of patients.[62]

Health information resource centers are designed to provide access to quality resources and support patient and family information gathering. Patient- and family-centered practices at the University of Washington Medical Center include involving patient and family advisers on their Health Information Resource Center committee to advise on policies, procedures, collection management, facility design, and operations. This committee guides Resource Center services that actively involve patients and their families in health information seeking, instruction on how to discern quality resources on the Web, and services that aid in coping with medical impacts on their daily lives. Collection management includes illustrations, education resources written at a variety of reading levels, advice on adding resources to address gaps in the collection, and use of plain language to enhance understanding. As in many health resource centers across the United States, patients and their families are encouraged to learn, ask questions, and be actively involved with their care team members in care planning and management.

Health Care and Adult Education Collaboration

As the extent of American adults' lack of basic health knowledge has become more widely known, health literacy advocates have sought opportunities to partner with health care providers and increase skill-building health literacy initiatives both within and at venues outside the health care sector. In recent years health professionals and adult educators have collaborated to develop health curriculum materials that can be incorporated into basic education lessons. An example is World Education's *Health and Literacy Compendium*. The collection contains health curricula designed for use in literacy settings, as well as literacy information and easy-to-read health materials for health professionals.[63]

The National Center for the Study of Adult Learning and Literacy has produced another resource—a series of curricula for adult educators to help students increase their health literacy skills.[64] The curricula include the following volumes:

- *Skills for Health Care Access and Navigation* addresses skills needed for accessing health-related services and for navigating health care systems.

- *Skills for Chronic Disease Management* addresses skills such as reading medicine labels, following directions, and measuring dosages correctly; using measurement tools to monitor health; monitoring symptoms and talking to health care professionals; and making critical decisions about health care.

- *Skills for Disease Prevention and Screening* addresses skills such as reading and interpreting risk communication materials, reading informed consent forms, understanding health information in the media, filling out forms, and discussing symptoms with a medical professional and making critical decisions about health care.

- *Health Literacy in Adult Basic Education: Designing Lessons, Units, and Evaluation Plans for an Integrated Curriculum* is designed to help adult educators develop health literacy units, lessons, and evaluation plans. It provides an overview of health literacy skills, offers templates for planning, and links to sample lessons from each of the above curriculum guides.

Collaboration between health care and adult education sectors can take other forms, such as referral of patients to adult education classes. For example, staff at Community Health Partners in Livingston, Montana, watch out for literacy red flags as part of their global assessment of patients' strengths and needs. Patients who are identified as having low literacy are asked if they wish to improve their reading and math skills. Clinicians refer, and often escort, interested patients to an on-site adult learning center. Preliminary data indicate that among persons with low literacy and symptoms of depression, adult basic literacy education as an adjunct to standard depression treatment increased patient self-efficacy and reduced depression symptoms.[65,66]

Transforming Health Care

Led by legislative, accreditation, and payer mandates as well as patients and families' voices, health care systems across the country are using a broad range of strategies to create error-free, safe health care environments. Transformation of care in health care organizations starts with an organizational assessment to identify opportunities for improvement; staff training and innovative programs integrate patients and families into the planning and implementation of patient safety initiatives.

Organizational Assessments

Organizational assessment tools have become an increasingly common way to measure an organization's strengths and to identify opportunities for improvement. Because assessment results often change organizational priorities, the content of the assessment and the processes used to conduct it are critical.

Currently there are a number of instruments that measure patient safety culture, health literacy, or patient- and family-centered care.[67,68,69,70,71] However, since the instruments used in each field were developed independently, these assessments do not draw on the strengths of the other fields. Organizational assessments need to triangulate so that health literacy and patient- and family-centered aspects of patient safety are measured.

Traditionally, organizational assessments are directed by health care administrators or clinicians and focus on collecting expert opinions. A few health literacy assessment tools have incorporated patients' views in the process. For example, *Health Literacy CAHPS®* and *Is Our Pharmacy Meeting Patients'*

Needs? A Pharmacy Health Literacy Assessment Tool both collect patient perspectives on their experience with care.[72,73] (See figure 5-5.) These tools use focus groups and patient surveys to collect patient perspectives on health literacy issues with patient safety implications.

Organizational assessments that evaluate patient- and family-centered policy, programs, and operations have gone a step further. Rather than only having the assessment done to or for them, patients and family members work with health care administrators and clinicians as part of the assessment team. For example, the Institute for Family-Centered Care has developed numerous health care self-assessment tools that recommend patient and family member participation on the assessment team.[74]

Figure 5-5. Health Literacy Organizational Assessments

Pharmacy Health Literacy Assessment Tool

Researchers at Emory University, Atlanta, under contract to the Agency for Healthcare Research and Quality, developed a three-part tool to assess the level of health literacy friendliness of pharmacies. Part 1 is completed by independent auditors who tour the pharmacy. Part 2 is a survey of pharmacy staff. Part 3 consists of focus groups with pharmacy patients to obtain their perceptions. Pharmacy patients are asked not only about the written information they receive from the pharmacy (e.g., pill bottle labels, consumer medical information) but also about the counseling they receive at the pharmacy. Patient perspectives are then triangulated with data from the other two sources to obtain an overall appraisal of the strengths and weaknesses of pharmacy operations.

Health Literacy CAHPS

A supplement to the Clinician/Group CAHPS, Health Literacy CAHPS is a survey that captures patients' health communication experiences at their doctor's office. Questions cover the transmission of both verbal and written health information, such as asking how often the doctor gave verbal, easy-to-understand instructions about how to take medicines and whether written information about how to take medicines was easy to understand. The instrument also asks about specific communication practices (e.g., using pictures or models, talking too fast, giving too much information), resulting in feedback that can be used for quality improvement. Health Literacy CAHPS is currently being field tested and is expected to be released soon by the Agency for Healthcare Research and Quality.

Patients and Families as Training Partners

Education and training have long been promoted as important measures for building a workforce equipped to tackle patient safety and health literacy. The Institute of Medicine recommends developing approaches to educating staff about patient safety,[75] and since early 2000, the Agency for Healthcare Research and Quality has been funding efforts to design and test "best practices," including a provider education focus to reduce errors. The Joint Commission's white paper on health literacy stresses the importance of patient-centered approaches to training health professionals.[76] Embracing patients and families as team members in training health care professionals is a powerful means to promote health literacy–sensitive approaches in patient safety policy and program development.

Patients and families can take on a variety of teaching roles in patient safety and health literacy curricula for health care practitioners (see figure 5-6).[77] Programs that have involved patients and families in training have identified many benefits. For example:

- Sharing of personal stories can help bring data to life.
- Patients and families improve clinician understanding of the toll of ambiguous or unclear terms and jargon and help to motivate teams to let go of "doing it one way because that's how we've always done it."
- Patients and families, through their observations in their care experience, notice more than we imagine. They can both validate and challenge professional assumptions about patient- and family-centered approaches to health literacy and patient safety.
- Allowing training participants to ask questions directly to patients and families both models patient- and family-centered care and eliminates the filter of the instructor's professional assumptions about the patient/family experience.

Figure 5-6.   Teaching Roles for Patients and Families in Health Literacy and Patient Safety Programs

- Sharing personal stories one-on-one or in a group setting
- Participating in small group discussions to train professionals
- Role-playing interactions with families
- Presenting at orientation meetings, grand rounds, and other continuing education programs
- Presenting at meetings and conferences
- Interacting with health professionals as patient advocates
- Co-instructing courses
- Consulting in curriculum development and review
- Participating in collaborative training projects
- Pairing with students to share patient and family care experiences over time
- Mentoring students who participate in service or other community learning projects
- Hosting students on home visits

Source: Adapted and reproduced with permission from "Creating Patient and Family Faculty Programs" (2007), Institute for Family-Centered Care, 7900 Wisconsin Ave., Suite 405, Bethesda, MD 20814; (301) 652-0281 (www.familycenteredcare.org).

Incorporating patients and family members into the training curriculum requires careful planning. Figure 5-7 lists the steps planners will want to take to ensure a training experience that is a success for both the patient/family faculty members and the trainees. Examples of trainings that have applied one or more of these patient- and family-centered planning strategies or curricula objectives and have engaged patient and family faculty in health literacy or patient safety training are highlighted below.

Iowa Health System Health Literacy Collaborative

The Iowa Health System, as part of its Health Literacy Collaborative conference, partnered with Iowa New Readers Coalition (a group of adult learners who have struggled with literacy and learning disabilities). New Readers provided constructive coaching and feedback on health professionals' communication skills during

Figure 5-7. Planning for Patient/Family Faculty

Selecting Patient/Family Participants in Training

Selection of advisers for participation in training involves securing names both through recommendations from staff and self-identification. Qualities of patients and families to involve are those who can share their story, give suggestions for improvement, and apply their experience to the bigger picture. Advisers recruited as trainers are often identified by clinicians who have relationships with their patients and families that welcome reflection on the care experience, and they are also often found in patients and families who have some experience serving as an adviser. From the selection step onward, it is important to demonstrate that your team values the adviser's time and contributions.

Preparing Patient/Family Participants

At the outset, you will want patients and family members, like all members of your training faculty, to know:

- Who will be at the training?
- What process will be followed?
- Who will be facilitating?
- What are the expectations regarding their participation?
- How can they best serve as teachers?
- Where will the training be held, and how long will it last?
- Is an honorarium available?
- Who can they turn to if they have any questions (a contact person)?

Preparing Staff

Preparations for staff involved in adviser partnerships in their trainings include:

- Affirm top-down commitment and expectations.
- Define patient/family faculty roles and responsibilities clearly to help staff know what to expect.
- Inform staff that patients and family members are committed to improving our care and systems.
- Keep abreast of any reluctance or even fear of patient/family involvement among trainees.

(Continued on next page)

Figure 5-7.   (Continued)

Debriefing Patient/Family Participants

Follow-up after the training with advisers as faculty is important and should include:

- Providing feedback on the training and about outcomes

- Identifying and addressing any ongoing support needs

- Communicating new and emerging patient safety issues at your health care facility

- Keeping the dialogue open—there is a vulnerability that comes with commitment to transparency

---

role-playing scenarios. New Readers also shared instructive stories of their health care challenges. For example, one woman said that after a colonoscopy she received discharge instructions she could not read. Not knowing she was supposed to rest after the procedure, she went to work and moved heavy boxes. That night she experienced significant, and totally preventable, pain.[78]

University of Virginia School of Medicine Integration of Health Literacy and Patient and Family as Faculty

Since 2000, the University of Virginia School of Medicine has been building patient-centered health literacy modules into existing courses throughout its four-year medical student and residency training. Approaches include lectures on health literacy, integration of literacy issues in case discussions, preceptor case write-ups that require at least one case with a health literacy focus, standardized patient cases with a health literacy focus for clinical performance exams, and involvement of patients with low literacy as faculty to demonstrate to the class effective communication skills. The University of Virginia School of Medicine has also developed a faculty development handbook of resources on health literacy to support and catalyze future faculty integration of health literacy into the curriculum. An increasing number of medical student and residency programs are incorporating health literacy training into their curricula.[79] Figure 5-8 is a list of tips to help build a health literacy curriculum into health professional training programs.

Figure 5-8. Tips for Building a Health Literacy Curriculum

1. Assess the health literacy of a sample of your patients to understand what the proportions of the various types of literacy are in your patient populations.

2. Review health literacy references in the literature and on credible Web sites. Contact those organizations that have resources for you to use. The Association of Standardized Patient Educators has health literacy cases available for free on a password-protected site for member organizations (http://www.aspeducators.org/).

3. Look for institutional, local, and state health literacy organizations in your area for local data, resources, and possible collaboration.

4. Actively involve patients and families as educators in a variety of roles and settings as an element of your curriculum. If you do not have a patient and family adviser program, recruit patients from an attending physician's panel of patients or involve new-reader members of local literacy organizations as faculty and/or codesigners of your curriculum.

Securing Support for Health Literacy in Your Health Care Profession Curriculum

1. *Get buy-in from leadership.* Dean (or highest level possible) and course director leadership is essential for adding credibility to your activities and for garnering support for adoption of your program.

2. *Find a champion who is widely connected.* This "connector" or "persuader" can be very helpful in identifying the key people to talk to and getting you resources and credibility.

3. *Prove the need at your health care organization.* Have some clear understanding of the patient literacy issues most commonly seen in your institution. For example, measure the literacy levels of patients provided care in one month for one high-volume clinical area. If you are able to make a financial impact case for the improvement in health literacy, you should do so. For example, show the costs of lost revenue in canceled or delayed surgical cases (the costs are even greater when the operating room sits unused during regular staffing hours) because of patient misunderstanding of their pre-op instructions.

4. *Insert the health literacy curricular thread.* Look at the existing courses in your institution and see where this information can go. Look for opportunities that allow you to weave repetition of the information and occasional "live" clinical examples. Focus on presenting a well-thought-out plan of action. When going to individual course directors, provide almost finished products—do most of the work for them, but allow them to put their own imprint on the elements.

5. *Create a health literacy faculty development and support handbook.* Develop a faculty development handbook on health literacy resources. Suggestions for resources to review when creating your handbook include:
   - The Joint Commission's *What Did the Doctor Say: Improving Health Literacy to Protect Patient Safety*[a]

(Continued on next page)

Figure 5-8. (Continued)

- The Institute of Medicine's *Health Literacy: A Prescription to End Confusion*[b]
- Abrams and colleagues' *Reducing the Risk by Designing a Safer, Shame-Free Health Care Environment*[c]
- The Agency for Healthcare Research and Quality's *Literacy and Health Outcomes*[d]
- Kutner and colleagues' *The Health Literacy of America's Adults: Results from the 2003 National Assessment of Adult Literacy*[e]
- The AMA Foundation's Health Literacy Kit, which includes a manual that is full of examples that can be used as teaching tools[f]
- Blaylock, Ahmann, and Johnson's "Creating Patient and Family Faculty Programs," Institute for Family-Centered Care[g]
- Institutional, local, and national health literacy resources
- Introductory lectures on health literacy with annotations, which help faculty applying threads in subsequent programs know the students' core content on health literacy
- Bibliography, sample cases, and hints about how to teach
- Annotated copy of the cases with discussion points, if using paper cases:
  — Include examples of patient and family education and information literature from your institution with annotations on why this is a good or poor example of literature.
  — Include copies of your institution's multidisciplinary care or patient education documentation forms or equivalent electronic medical record areas referring to learning needs assessment and patient understanding after instruction, clearly marked.

---

[a] Joint Commission, *What Did the Doctor Say? Improving Health Literacy to Protect Patient Safety* (Oakbrook Terrace, IL: Joint Commission, 2007).

[b] Institute of Medicine, *Health Literacy: A Prescription to End Confusion* (Washington, DC: National Academies Press, 2004).

[c] M. A. Abrams, L. L. Hung, A. B. Kashuba, J. G. Schwartzberg, P. E. Sokol, and K. C. Vergara, *Reducing the Risk by Designing a Safer, Shame-Free Health Care Environment* (Chicago: American Medical Association Foundation, 2007).

[d] N. D. Berkman, D. A. DeWalt, M. P. Pignone, S. L. Sheridan, K. N. Lohr, S. F. Sutton, T. Swinson, and A. J. Bonito, *Literacy and Health Outcomes, Evidence Report Technology Assessment* (Rockville, MD: Agency for Healthcare Research and Quality, 2004) [www.ahrq.gov/clinic/epcsums/litsum.htm].

[e] M. Kutner, E. Greenberg, Y. Jin, C. Paulsen, and S. White, *The Health Literacy of America's Adults: Results from the 2003 National Assessment of Adult Literacy* (Washington, DC: National Center for Educational Statistics, 2006).

[f] American Medical Association, *Health Literacy Introductory Kit* (Chicago: American Medical Association Foundation, 1999) [www.amafoundation.org].

[g] B. Blaylock, E. Ahmann, and B. H. Johnson, "Creating Patient and Family Faculty Programs" (Bethesda, MD: Institute for Family-Centered Care, 2002) [www.familycenteredcare.org].

Source: Adapted with permission from Dr. Claudette Dalton, MD, American Association of Medical Colleges Poster Presentation, "Initiating a Health Literacy Curriculum," November 2003.

Lucille Packard Children's Hospital at Stanford— Family-Centered Approaches to Disclose Errors

Lucille Packard Children's Hospital recently completed a pilot study that used technology to simulate real-life error scenarios for nurses to practice disclosure of medical error. Families helped create the training scenarios, acted in the simulations, and provided feedback to the nurses. The study showed a significant increase in nurses' communication self-efficacy when using a family-centered approach to disclose errors. Nurse trainees gave family involvement the highest rating (94 percent) of all training components.[80]

Broadening Team Membership to Include Patients and Families

Patients and families are beginning to participate at the policy and planning levels of patient safety improvements. Innovations include bringing in patient and family advisers as members of health care systems' patient safety committees and task forces focusing on priority safety initiatives. The University of Washington Medical Center, Dana-Farber Cancer Institute, and Johns Hopkins Medical Center are a few of the growing number of health care systems that welcome patients and family members on their patient safety committees to inform and influence patient safety policy and program development.

For example, patients, family members, and clinicians at Dana-Farber Cancer Institute codesigned and participate in patient safety liaison rounds. Trained patient and family advisory council members assess current patients' and families' knowledge of important safety practices and elicit their quality and safety concerns. For example, advisers trained as patient safety liaisons ask:

- Have you experienced anything today or in the recent past that you would perceive as unsafe within your plan of care?

- Do you know what medications you take and what their side effects are?

The concerns identified in these patient-to-patient interviews have yielded useful information about specific safety and quality lapses and have led to numerous improvements and a safer patient care environment.[81] Dana-Farber has published a tool kit for other health care organizations to implement the patient safety liaison program. The tool kit includes organizational readiness assessment tools, program guidelines, training materials, and implementation and evaluation tools to support successful adoption.[82]

Vanderbilt Medical Center, Nashville, Tennessee, also pairs patients and family members with their leadership-led quality and safety walking rounds for inpatient care. Codesigned with patients and their families, the program involves leadership interviewing staff to capture their suggestions on how to make sure systems that support safe practices are in place. The successes of having patients and family members participate in inpatient rounds have inspired plans to expand patient and family member involvement in leadership rounds to outpatient care.

Winnipeg Regional Health Authority in Manitoba, Canada provides another example of bringing patients and family members into the decision-making process.[83] Its Patient Safety Patient and Family Advisory Council directly involves patients and their families in its Regional Integrated Patient Safety Strategy. The council has explored policy issues such as patient access to medical records and patient designation of family/ friends as health care proxies/representatives.

Health Literacy Implications of Patient Safety Partnering

Including patients and family members in efforts to improve health care safety will change the dynamics of patient safety activities. Verbal interactions at meetings or on rounds will have to change to accommodate the patient/family participant. Medical professionals frequently use technical terms that are confusing to persons not in the health care profession. Health care institutions often use acronyms that constitute a nonsensical alphabet soup to anyone who isn't an insider. Health care organizations that want to genuinely collaborate with patients and families must realize that jargon can get in the way of their understanding and contributing. Entrenched communication patterns, however, are hard to change. Figure 5-9 lists some suggestions of how to reduce jargon in verbal interactions.

Figure 5-9. Reducing Jargon

There are many approaches staff can use to help limit the use of jargon and acronyms when speaking with patients and families.

- Make up a "jargon list" of the medical phrases and jargon you hear others using. Then develop a list of alternative words. For example, say "high blood pressure" instead of "hypertension" and "heart" instead of "cardiac."

- If you catch yourself using jargon, stop and choose new words. When introducing medical terms to explain diagnostic and treatment choices, provide explanations of the medical terms the first time you use them.

- If you catch others using jargon, ask them to explain in plain language in a noncritical tone.

- Don't assume everyone knows terms that are commonly used in health care. If you can't avoid using a medical term, be sure you define it in plain language.

- Avoid or limit use of acronyms. Always explain the acronym. Then ask patients if they are OK with using the acronym.

- Ask yourself how a nonspecialist would describe the same idea. Try explaining concepts and terms using a conversational tone.

- When you are in committee meetings with patients or family members, define terms the first time they are used. For committees or councils that have patient and family membership, ask your patient and family membership if they would work with staff to create a glossary and acronym reference list that can then be distributed as part of orientation packets for new patient and family members.

- Ask facilitators of meetings with patients or family members to create a respectful environment in which everyone can ask for terms or acronyms to be defined or explained, if needed.

Source: University of Michigan, *Simplification Guide to Medical Terms* (Ann Arbor, MI: University of Michigan Medical School Institutional Review Board, 1999).

In addition to reducing the use of jargon, it is also important to clarify what important background knowledge of health and health systems concepts would be helpful to include in new committee members' orientation, especially patient and family members. Routinely providing explanations for new concepts as they are applied in team discussions is helpful, and creating an atmosphere in which questions are encouraged can foster an environment where patients, families, and clinicians alike feel they are an integral part of the team. Pairing new patient and family advisers with an experienced adviser or staff member of the committee/team for the first quarter of their tenure for either pre- or postmeeting consultation can serve to clarify organizational references, discreetly address questions, and strengthen participation.

Patient safety activities that require reading and writing skills call for sensitivity. Patient and family team members may not want to admit that they are unable to complete these tasks. Consider heterogeneous groupings for such assignments, coupling patients and family members with health care professionals. Encourage the leader of patient safety activities to mention the key concepts in required readings as an introduction to discussion.

Directions for patients and families, such as when to activate a rapid response team or how to review a brochure, should be built into any plan to make them integral members of the patient safety team. This is especially critical when patients and families have limited health literacy or are unfamiliar with the Western health care system. While perhaps harder to recruit, diverse patients and families—both in terms of ethnicity and health literacy—engaged in the patient safety enterprise will result in patient and family guidance that is truly representative of the patient population.

Link Health Literacy with Patient Safety Initiatives

Effective communication is central to providing a care experience that is safe, supports patient and family collaboration, and promotes understanding and shared decision making. As well as developing new technologies for improving patient safety, we need to strengthen communication that actively engages health care providers, patients, and their families as partners in pursuit of safe, high-quality care.

Health care systems across the United States are innovating and applying health literacy precepts to strategies that support patient and family partnership to improve the safety of care. The evidence base, however, lags behind practice. There are few studies of the effectiveness of health literacy interventions or initiatives aimed at engaging individuals in clinical care to improve patient safety.[84,85] But the strong association of health literacy with health outcomes and the correlation of patient participation and patient-centered care with outcomes and satisfaction give credence to the contention that both must function as drivers of safe care.[86,87,88,89]

Health care organizations, funders, and policy makers need to consider how to support further innovations and research. The recent merger of the Partnership for Clear Health Communication, a health literacy organization, with the National Patient Safety Foundation has potential to further the integration of health literacy and communication techniques with patient safety initiatives.

While synthesis of health literacy and patient and family involvement in all patient safety activities is the ideal, incremental changes are also powerful. Even small steps move us toward our goals of changing and improving the clinician, patient, and family experience and building the safest health care systems possible. We hope that this chapter clarifies how patient- and family-centered care approaches to patient safety and health literacy improve health care delivery and ultimately create optimal safe care experiences for clinicians, patients, and their families.

The organization's leaders must determine progress in implementing patient and family partnerships in health literacy and patient safety initiatives. These leaders set the tone and define the boundaries on permissible innovation. Clinicians and staff members can lead by taking advantage of every opportunity to involve patients and families in designing patient safety, health literacy, and patient- and family-centered care practices. Patients and family members need to be invited and supported as they become leaders as well, and to be welcomed as valuable members of patient safety teams.

References

1. Institute of Medicine, *Health Literacy: A Prescription to End Confusion* (Washington, DC: National Academies Press, 2004).
2. M. A. Abrams, L. L. Hung, A. B. Kashuba, J. G. Schwartzberg, P. E. Sokol, and K. C. Vergara, *Reducing the Risk by Designing a Safer, Shame-Free Health Care Environment* (Chicago: American Medical Association Foundation, 2007); Joint Commission, *What Did the Doctor Say? Improving Health Literacy to Protect Patient Safety* (Oakbrook Terrace, IL: Joint Commission, 2007).
3. Joint Commission, *What Did the Doctor Say,* 6.
4. U.S. Department of Health and Human Services, *Healthy People 2010: Understanding and Improving Health* (Washington, DC: U.S. Government Printing Office, 2000).
5. D. W. Baker, "The Meaning and the Measure of Health Literacy," *Journal of General Internal Medicine* 21, no. 8 (2006): 878–83.
6. D. P. Andrulis and C. Brach, "Integrating Literacy, Culture, and Language to Improve Health Care Quality for Diverse Populations," *American Journal of Health Behavior* 31, suppl. 1 (2007): S122–S133.
7. Baker, "The Meaning and the Measure of Health Literacy."
8. M. Kutner, E. Greenberg, Y. Jin, C. Paulsen, and S. White, *The Health Literacy of America's Adults: Results from the 2003 National Assessment of Adult Literacy* (Washington, DC: National Center for Educational Statistics, 2006).
9. N. D. Berkman, D. A. DeWalt, M. P. Pignone, S. L. Sheridan, K. N. Lohr, S. F. Sutton, T. Swinson, and A. J. Bonito, *Literacy and Health Outcomes, Evidence Report Technology Assessment* (Rockville, MD: Agency for Healthcare Research and Quality, 2004).
10. B. D. Weiss, *Health Literacy: A Manual for Clinicians* (Chicago: American Medical Association Foundation and American Medical Association, 2003).
11. A. Coulter and J. Ellins, "Effectiveness of Strategies for Informing, Educating, and Involving Patients," *British Medical Journal* 335, no. 7609 (2007) 24–27.

12. Weiss, *Health Literacy: A Manual for Clinicians.*
13. A. Kleinman, L. Eisenberg, and B. Good, "Culture, Illness, and Care: Clinical Lessons from Anthropologic and Cross-Cultural Research," *Annals of Internal Medicine* 88, no. 2 (1978): 251–58.
14. R. A. Bell, R. L. Kravitz, D. Thom, E. Krupat, and R. Azari, "Unsaid but Not Forgotten: Patients' Unvoiced Desires in Office Visits," *Archives of Internal Medicine* 161, no. 16 (2001): 1977–84.
15. J. Schneider, S. H. Kaplan, S. Greenfield, W. Li, and I. B. Wilson, "Better Physician-Patient Relationships Are Associated with Higher Reported Adherence to Antiretroviral Therapy in Patients with HIV Infection," *Journal of General Internal Medicine* 19, no. 11 (2004): 1096–1103.
16. M. M. Ward, S. Sundaramurthy, D. Lotstein, T. M. Bush, C. M. Neuwelt, and R. L. Street, Jr., "Participatory Patient-Physician Communication and Morbidity in Patients with Systemic Lupus Erythematosus," *Arthritis Rheum* 49, no. 6 (2003): 810–18.
17. Partnership for Clear Health Communication, "Ask Me 3" (North Adams, MA: Partnership for Clear Health Communication) [www.npsf.org/askme3]. Accessed August 21, 2007.
18. Agency for Healthcare Research and Quality, "Questions Are the Answer" (Rockville, MD: AHRQ) [www.ahrq.gov/questionsarethe answer]. Accessed August 23, 2007.
19. Coulter and Ellins, "Effectiveness of Strategies for Informing, Educating, and Involving Patients."
20. Institute of Medicine, *Health Literacy: A Prescription to End Confusion* (Washington, DC: National Academies Press, 2004).
21. P. E. Austin, R. Matlack II, K. A. Dunn, C. Kesler, and C. K. Brown, "Discharge Instructions: Do Illustrations Help Our Patients Understand Them?" *Annals of Emergency Medicine* 25, no. 3 (1995): 317–20.
22. C. Delp and J. Jones, "Communicating Information to Patients: The Use of Cartoon Illustrations to Improve Comprehension of Instructions," *Academy of Emergency Medicine* 3, no. 3 (1996): 264–70.
23. L. Cooper-Patrick, J. J. Gallo, J. J. Gonzales, H. T. Vu, N. R. Powe, C. Nelson, and D. E. Ford, "Race, Gender, and Partnership in the Patient-Physician Relationship," *Journal of the American Medical Association* 282, no. 6 (1999): 583–89.
24. C. C. Doak, L. G. Doak, and J. H. Root, *Teaching Patients with Low Literacy Skills,* 2nd ed. (Philadelphia, PA: J. B. Lippincott Company, 1996).
25. Ibid.
26. P. Lane, M. Blanco, L. Ford, and H. Smith Mirenda, *The Health Literacy Style Manual* (Reston, VA: Maximus Center for Health Literacy, 2005).

27. National Resource Center for Health Information Technology, "Accessible Health Information Technology (HIT) for Limited-Literacy Populations: Checklist for Developers and Purchasers of HII," (Rockville, MD: Agency for Healthcare Research and Quality, 2007).

28. E. Peters, J. Hibbard, P. Slovic, and N. Dieckmann, "Numeracy Skill and the Communication, Comprehension, and Use of Risk-Benefit Information," *Health Affairs (Millwood)* 26, no. 3 (2007): 741–48.

29. Institute of Medicine, *Preventing Medication Errors* (Washington, DC: National Academies Press, 2006).

30. Weiss, *Health Literacy: A Manual for Clinicians.*

31. M. V. Williams, T. Davis, R. M. Parker, and B. D. Weiss, "The Role of Health Literacy in Patient-Physician Communication," *Family Medicine* 34, no. 5 (2002): 383–89.

32. Weiss, *Health Literacy: A Manual for Clinicians.*

33. B. D. Weiss, M. Z. Mays, W. Martz, K. M. Castro, D. A. DeWalt, M. P. Pignone, J. Mockbee, and F. A. Hale, "Quick Assessment of Literacy in Primary Care: The Newest Vital Sign," *Annals of Family Medicine* 3, no. 6 (2005): 514–22.

34. N. S. Parikh, R. M. Parker, J. R. Nurss, D. W. Baker, and M. V. Williams, "Shame and Health Literacy: The Unspoken Connection," *Patient Education and Counseling* 27, no. 1 (1996): 33–39.

35. D. W. Baker, R. M. Parker, M. V. Williams, K. Pitkin, N. S. Parikh, W. Coates, and M. Imara, "The Health Care Experience of Patients with Low Literacy," *Archives of Family Medicine* 5, no. 6 (1996): 329–34; H. Osborne, "In Other Words: Healthcare Communication from an Adult Learner's Perspective," *Boston Globe's On Call Magazine,* April 2004 [www.healthliteracy.com/article.asp?PageID=3749].

36. Osborne, "In Other Words."

37. J. G. Ryan, F. Leuguen, B. D. Weiss, S. Albury, T. Jennings, F. Velez, and N. Salibi, "Will Patients Agree to Have Their Literacy Skills Assessed in Clinical Practice?" *Health Education Research* (epub ahead of print, September 22, 2007).

38. Weiss, *Health Literacy: A Manual for Clinicians.*

39. M. K. Paasche-Orlow, D. Schillinger, S. M. Greene, and E. H. Wagner, "How Health Care Systems Can Begin to Address the Challenge of Limited Literacy," *Journal of General Internal Medicine* 21, no. 8 (2006): 884–87.

40. R. M. Parker, T. C. Davis, and M. V. Williams, "Patients with Limited Health Literacy," in *Patient and Family Education in Managed Care,* W. B. Bateman, ed. (New York: Springer, 1999).

41. P. F. Bass, III, J. F. Wilson, C. H. Griffith, and D. R. Barnett, "Residents' Ability to Identify Patients with Poor Literacy Skills," *Academic Medicine* 77, no. 10 (2002): 1039–41.

42. Laurie Francis, executive director, Community Health Partners, Livingston, MT, interview with author, September 10, 2007.

43. S. Kripalani, L. E. Henderson, E. Y. Chiu, R. Robertson, P. Kolm, and T. A. Jacobson, "Predictors of Medication Self-Management Skill in a Low-Literacy Population," *Journal of General Internal Medicine* 21, no. 8 (2006): 852–56.

44. National Quality Forum, *Improving Patient Safety through Informed Consent for Patients with Limited Health Literacy: An Implementation Report* (Washington, DC: National Quality Forum, 2005).

45. C. A. Mancuso and M. Rincon, "Impact of Health Literacy on Longitudinal Asthma Outcomes," *Journal of General Internal Medicine* 21, no. 8 (2006): 813–17.

46. T. K. Gandhi, S. N. Weingart, J. Borus, A. C. Seger, J. Peterson, E. Burdick, D. L. Seger, K. Shu, F. Federico, L. L. Leape, and D. W. Bates, "Adverse Drug Events in Ambulatory Care," *New England Journal of Medicine* 348, no. 16 (2003): 1556–64.

47. T. C. Davis, M. S. Wolf, P. F. Bass III, J. A. Thompson, H. H. Tilson, M. Neuberger, and R. M. Parker, "Literacy and Misunderstanding Prescription Drug Labels," *Annals of Internal Medicine* 145, no. 12 (2006): 887–94.

48. D. Schillinger, E. Machtinger, F. Wang, M. Rodriguez, and A. Bindman, "Preventing Medication Errors in Ambulatory Care: The Importance of Establishing Regimen Concordance," in *Advances in Patient Safety: From Research to Implementation* (Rockville, MD: Agency for Healthcare Research and Quality, 2005).

49. A. Nathan, L. Goodyear, A. Lovejoy, and I. Savage, "Patients' Views of the Value of 'Brown Bag' Medication Reviews," *International Journal of Pharmacy Practice* 8 (2000): 298–304.

50. Ohio Patient Safety Institute, "Brown Bag Toolkit" (Columbus, OH: Ohio Patient Safety Institute) [www.ohiopatientsafety.org/meds/default.htm]. Accessed September 6, 2007.

51. Joint Commission, *Medication Reconciliation Handbook* (Oakbrook Terrace, IL: Joint Commission Resources, 2006).

52. M. Daniel and J. M. Langle, "Partnering with Families to Improve Patient Safety with Lean Processing," paper presented at the Third International Conference on Patient- and Family-Centered Care, Seattle, WA, July 2007.

53. National Quality Forum, *Improving Patient Safety through Informed Consent for Patients with Limited Health Literacy*, 1.

54. National Quality Forum, *Serious Reportable Events in Healthcare: A Consensus Report* (Washington, DC: National Quality Forum, 2002).

55. C. H. Braddock, III, K. A. Edwards, N. M. Hasenberg, T. L. Laidley, and W. Levinson, "Informed Decision Making in Outpatient Practice: Time to Get Back to Basics," *Journal of the American Medical Association* 282, no. 24 (1999): 2313–20.

56. P. Graham, "Type of Consent Does Not Influence Patient Recall of Serious Potential Radiation Toxicity of Adjuvant Breast Radiotherapy," *Australasia Radiology* 47, no. 4 (2003): 416–21.

57. J. H. Bergler, A. C. Pennington, M. Metcalfe, and E. D. Freis, "Informed Consent: How Much Does the Patient Understand?" *Clinical Pharmacology Therapeutics* 27, no. 4 (1980): 435–40.

58. B. Vardigan, "Illiteracy: A Hidden Health Hazard," *Consumer Health Interactive,* May 29 2007 [http://healthresources.caremark .com/topic/healthliteracy]. Accessed September 6, 2007.

59. National Quality Forum, *Implementing a National Voluntary Consensus Standard for Informed Consent: A User's Guide for Healthcare Professionals* (Washington, DC: National Quality Forum, 2005).

60. E. H. Wagner, "The Chronic Care Model" [http://www.improving chroniccare.org/change/model/components.html]. Accessed December 24, 2007.

61. K. R. Lorig, D. S. Sobel, P. L. Ritter, D. Laurent, and M. Hobbs, "Effect of a Self-Management Program on Patients with Chronic Disease," *Effective Clinical Practice* 4, no. 6 (2001): 256–62.

62. L. Sweeney, A. Halpert, and J. Waranoff, "Patient-Centered Management of Complex Patients Can Reduce Costs Without Shortening Life," *American Journal of Managed Care* 13, no. 2 (2007): 84–92.

63. World Education, *Health and Literacy Compendium: An Annotated Bibliography of Print and Web-Based Health Materials for Use with Limited-Literacy Adults* (Boston: World Education) [http://health literacy.worlded.org/]. Accessed September 11, 2007.

64. Harvard School of Public Health, Health Literacy Studies, "Health Literacy Curricula" (Boston: Harvard School of Public Health, Health Literacy Studies) [www.hsph.harvard.edu/healthliteracy/ curricula.html]. Accessed August 12, 2007.

65. L. Francis, B. D. Weiss, J. H. Senf, K. Heist, and R. Hargraves, "Does Literacy Education Improve Symptoms of Depression and Self-Efficacy in Individuals with Low Literacy and Depressive Symptoms? A Preliminary Investigation," *Journal of the American Board of Family Medicine* 20, no. 1 (2007): 23–27.

66. B. D. Weiss, L. Francis, J. H. Senf, K. Heist, and R. Hargraves, "Literacy Education as Treatment for Depression in Patients with Limited Literacy and Depression: A Randomized Controlled Trial," *Journal of General Internal Medicine* 21, no. 8 (2006): 823–28.

67. Agency for Healthcare Research and Quality, "Patient Safety Culture Surveys" (Rockville, MD: AHRQ) [http://www.ahrq.gov/ qual/hospculture/]. Accessed August 20, 2007.

68. University of Texas Center of Excellence for Patient Safety Research and Practice, "Safety Attitudes Questionnaire and Safety Climate Survey" (Houston, TX: University of Texas Center of Excellence) [www.uth.tmc.edu/schools/med/imed/patient_safety/survey&tools. html]. Accessed September 22, 2007.

69. S. J. Singer, D. M. Gaba, J. J. Geppert, A. D. Sinaiko, S. K. Howard, and K. C. Park, "The Culture of Safety: Results of an Organization-Wide Survey in 15 California Hospitals," *Quality and Safety in Health Care* 12, no. 2 (2003): 112–18.

70. R. E. Rudd and J. E. Anderson, *The Health Literacy Environment of Hospitals and Health Centers. Partners for Action: Making Your Healthcare Facility Literacy-Friendly* (Boston: National Center for the Study of Adult Learning and Literacy and Health and Adult Literacy and Learning Initiative, Harvard School of Public Health, 2006).

71. Institute for Family-Centered Care, *Patient- and Family-Centered Care: A Hospital Self-Assessment Inventory* (Bethesda, MD: Institute for Family-Centered Care) [http://www.aha.org/aha/content/2005/pdf/assessment.pdf]. Accessed August 15, 2007.

72. Agency for Healthcare Research and Quality, "CAHPS Health Literacy Item Set" (Rockville, MD: Agency for Healthcare Research and Quality) [www.cahps.ahrq.gov/content/products/HL/PROD_HL_Intro.asp]. Accessed August 15, 2007.

73. K. L. Jacobson, J. A. Gazmarian, S. Kripilani, K. J. McMorris, S. C. Blake, and C. Brach, *Is Our Pharmacy Meeting Patients' Needs? A Pharmacy Health Literacy Assessment Tool. User's Guide* (Rockville, MD: Agency for Healthcare Research and Quality, 2007).

74. Institute for Family-Centered Care, *Patient- and Family-Centered Care: A Hospital Self-Assessment Inventory.*

75. Institute of Medicine, *To Err Is Human: Building a Safer Health System* (Washington, DC: National Academies Press, 2000).

76. Joint Commission, *What Did the Doctor Say?*

77. B. Blaylock, E. Ahmann, and B. H. Johnson, "Creating Patient and Family Faculty Programs" (Bethesda, MD: Institute for Family-Centered Care, 2002).

78. Norma Kenoyer, remarks at the Iowa Health System Health Literacy Collaborative–Iowa New Readers Coalition joint conference, April 13, 2007.

79. S. Kripilani, K. L. Jacoson, S. Brown, K. Manning, K. J. Rask, and T. A. Jacobson, "Development and Implementation of a Health Literacy Training Program for Medical Residents," *Medical Education Online* 11, no. 13 (2006): 1–8.

80. J. Conway, B. Johnson, S. Edgman-Levitan, J. Schlucter, D. Ford, P. Sodomka, and L. Simmons, *Partnering with Patients and Families to Design a Patient and Family-Centered Health Care System* (Bethesda, MD: Institute for Family-Centered Care, 2007).

81. S. N. Weingart, J. Price, D. Duncombe, M. Connor, K. Sommer, K. A. Conley, B. E. Bierer, and P. R. Ponte, "Patient-Reported Safety and Quality of Care in Outpatient Oncology," *Joint Commission Journal of Quality and Patient Safety* 33, no. 2 (2007): 83–94.

82. Dana-Farber Cancer Institute, "Patient Safety Rounding Toolkit" (Boston: Dana Farber Cancer Institute) [www.dana-farber.org/pat/patient-safety/patient-safety-resources/]. Accessed August 29, 2007.

83. Winnipeg Regional Health Authority, "Regional Integrated Patient Safety Strategy" (Winnipeg, MB) [http://www.wrha.mb.ca/health-info/patientsafety/ripss.php]. Accessed August 21, 2007.

84. Berkman et al., *Literacy and Health Outcomes, Evidence Report Technology Assessment.*

85. Coulter and Ellins, "Effectiveness of Strategies for Informing, Educating, and Involving Patients."

86. K. Fiscella, S. Meldrum, P. Franks, C. G. Shields, P. Duberstein, S. H. McDaniel, and R. M. Epstein, "Patient Trust: Is It Related to Patient-Centered Behavior of Primary Care Physicians?" *Medical Care* 42, no. 11 (2004): 1049–55.

87. S. A. Flocke, W. L. Miller, and B. F. Crabtree, "Relationships between Physician Practice Style, Patient Satisfaction, and Attributes of Primary Care," *Journal of Family Practice* 51, no. 10 (2002): 495–98.

88. Cooper-Patrick et al., "Race, Gender, and Partnership in the Patient-Physician Relationship."

89. M. Stewart, J. B. Brown, A. Donner, I. R. McWhinney, J. Oates, W. W. Weston, and J. Jordan, "The Impact of Patient-Centered Care on Outcomes," *Journal of Family Practice* 49, no. 9 (2000): 796–804.

6

Enabling Patient Involvement without Increasing Liability Risks

*James W. Saxton, Esquire,
and Maggie M. Finkelstein, Esquire*

Before coming to the hospital tomorrow morning, use this pen to mark "No" on the knee that I won't be operating on and "Yes" on the knee I will be operating on. That way we'll be sure to operate on the knee that's giving you problems.

Please help remind us to wash our hands before we perform any hands-on procedures. We don't want to spread infections, and hand washing is an important preventive measure.

If at any time during your hospital stay you don't feel safe or have a concern about the care you are receiving, here is the phone number of a person whom you or your family can contact.

If one of the complications occurs, and, as I explained they are remote, please come back to me so we can review what has occurred and I can answer all your questions.

Physicians, nurses, other caregivers, and organizations are reaching out to patients to encourage them to become active participants in the patient's health care experience. The advancement of safer health care services can be accomplished in part by patient involvement in their own care and effective collaboration with caregivers. Requesting that patients notify the physician or staff members of perceived mistakes or unsafe situations could ultimately lead to a reduction of adverse events.[1] An example of engaging the patient in error reduction is in prevention of wrong-site surgery. The patient (or a family member) can be

163

actively involved in the surgery site identification process. There are many other health care situations in which the patient may be able to recognize and prevent errors from occurring.

Regrettably, patients are often an untapped resource when it comes to safeguarding health care services. They need to become true members of the health care team before, during, and after treatment. Several factors affect this lack of patient involvement, perhaps the most pervasive being the traditional "lone hero" model of the medical profession, which can limit the openness and equality of caregiver-patient interactions.[2] This traditional model conflicts with the contemporary values of many patients who are seeking a more collaborative and partnering relationship with practitioners. Physicians and other caregivers must learn how to create legitimate opportunities for patients to be involved in making health care safer and to give them the tools (i.e., knowledge and skills) to be effective safety partners. Numerous suggestions on how this can be accomplished are found throughout this book. This chapter focuses on improving physician-patient communication, both preintervention and postintervention, which can lead to better patient outcomes and both a reduction in the potential of a professional liability claim and the severity of that claim if pursued.

Benefits of Patient Involvement

Practicing true patient involvement and improving communication between patients and their health care providers have numerous beneficial effects. These practices increase patient satisfaction and strengthen mutual trust. Open lines of communication can also help keep patients' expectations in line with reality. All of these benefits can lead to a decrease in professional liability lawsuits as well as a decrease in medical errors.[3]

Culturally, a significant change is needed in our approach to sharing information with patients and their families, both in disclosing relevant information prior to treatment and in disclosing adverse events and medical errors after they occur.

One study in 2000 revealed that physicians were not eager to acknowledge or discuss medical errors for various reasons, including threats of medical malpractice lawsuits, concerns about personal reputation and job security, and the potential for punitive actions by licensing boards.[4]

Clearly, physicians, staff members, and risk managers have been concerned about disclosure of medical error and its legal implications, but given the current professional liability landscape, which has progressed since 2004, when this chapter was first published in an earlier book, disclosure can be a very positive risk reduction measure. Such measures have taken on greater importance in this new environment.

Pay-for-performance initiatives are continuing to grow, and transparency in health care is taking on much greater significance. Malpractice claims are often triggered by the coupling of an adverse outcome with an aggravating circumstance such as inadequate documentation, service lapses, and miscommunications. Further, failure to disclose an adverse outcome or medical error is actually being used by plaintiffs as a basis for the imposition of punitive damages and large verdict awards. When information sharing is done right—the right way, at the right time, by the right people—the potential for litigation and large verdicts can be reduced.

Disclosure and Information Sharing

Within the context of this chapter, the term *disclosure* is used to describe communications in which the practitioner reveals medical errors, complications, or near misses that occur after the fact. Practitioner partnering with a patient applies to informed consent discussions on the risks of treatment as well as general information sharing. We do not suggest that the legal standard for informed consent be changed, only that the information sharing process be enhanced to achieve possible safety benefits for the patient and the caregiver. Throughout this chapter, the terms *disclosure* and *information sharing* are used synonymously.

Disclosure, or sharing of medical information with patients, has cultural, legal, and regulatory implications and considerations. A health care professional's fear of a lawsuit may actually create barriers to effective practitioner-patient partnerships. Sometimes, health care professionals feel that less information sharing is actually better. In other words, providing less information to the patient can prevent patient anxiety and a stressful environment. However, at times, the opposite is true. Involving patients in their own care and providing them with an understanding of the care can often lead to positive results in outcomes and enable a more effective communication environment, particularly should an adverse outcome occur. As always, caregivers must strike the right balance between withholding and sharing information with patients—it is truly fact specific.

When it comes to disclosure of an actual medical error, one study suggests that doctors are clearly worried that admitting mistakes can make a lawsuit more likely.[5] This type of attitude can inhibit physicians and other caregivers from suggesting to patients that a mistake might happen in the first place. Medicine is not an exact science, and bringing patient expectations in line with reality can help your cause, not hinder it.

Even though studies have repeatedly shown that most medical errors are caused by faulty systems, not people, it is common for practitioners to view mistakes as personal failures.[6] Operating from this belief, it is reasonable for caregivers to deduce that they will be held personally liable should a mistake actually happen. Thus, physicians and other caregivers may be reluctant to engage patients as partners in preventing errors if such interactions are thought to increase the risk of liability lawsuits. However, early results, discussed later in this chapter, reveal that disclosure done in the right way by the right people can reduce lawsuit frequency and severity.

Admittedly, the threat of a lawsuit can never be completely eliminated, but many of the liability fears associated with frank and complete practitioner-patient dialogue are overstated. By communicating more effectively with patients, practitioners can enhance a patient's health care. Open, honest, and compassionate interactions can help patients understand that they are an important part of the health care team—one in which all team members are trying their best to achieve the best outcomes.

Most medical errors do not occur because of incompetent or reckless individuals, substandard care, malpractice, or even deliberate mistakes; errors may occur even when the medical care is optimal. Health care is a complex sociotechnological industry and, as with other complex industries, there is a high potential for error.[7] It would be unfortunate if the fear of professional liability lawsuits holds health care professionals back from enlisting help from patients (and their family members) in error prevention. Another "set of eyes" should be a welcome safeguard in the health care system. Patients are an untapped resource.

In November 1999, the National Academy of Science's Institute of Medicine released a controversial report that purported to show, for the first time, the extent to which medical errors may cause preventable deaths in the United States. The report estimated that between 44,000 and 98,000 Americans die each year because of medical errors.[8] Even though medical errors may rank as the eighth leading cause of death, true patient collaboration has the potential for improving the detection and prevention of such errors. At the same time, legal issues appear to inhibit effective practitioner-patient partnerships. A better understanding of these legal issues can help physicians, nurses, and other caregivers put to rest some of their fears. Even legal barriers that are both real and significant are not insurmountable. Practitioners can provide a patient with information about his or her own care, including the potential for errors and adverse outcomes, without an increased risk of a lawsuit. Research data have shown that disclosure reduces both the frequency and severity of claims.[9]

The legal questions related to disclosure fall into two categories: information sharing about the potential for medical errors (preintervention) and information sharing following the occurrence of an incident or medical error (postintervention).

Following is a discussion of the liability fears that accompany disclosure in these two categories, together with recommendations for how these fears can be confronted and reduced.

Preintervention Communication

The pursuit of safer health care services can be advanced by patients' involvement in their own care, better communication between practitioners and patients, and inclusion of patients as partners on the health care team. The effects of practicing true patient involvement and increasing practitioner-patient communication are beneficial in many ways. They increase patient satisfaction and strengthen the bond between the clinician and the patient. As a result, patients are more likely to follow the recommended course of treatment. Open lines of communication also keep patients' expectations in line with reality. All of these benefits lead to a decrease in professional liability lawsuits as well as a decrease in medical errors.[10] There are two aspects of preintervention communication: (1) general information sharing, enhanced by family-centered care and (2) the informed consent process.

General Information Sharing

Patients may be in the best position to watch for medical errors, and for this reason patients may be one of our most underutilized safety resources. The patient has the personal incentive for a positive outcome and may be the most aware of his or her health and the needs associated with treatment. It only makes sense, then, for practitioners to partner with patients. Some of the measures intended to reinforce the practitioner-patient relationship as a team effort include the following:

- Requesting that patients notify physicians or staff members of any treatment mistakes or errors
- Encouraging patients to be more accountable for their own health[11]

Another useful patient-practitioner collaboration tool that is gaining popularity is a patient journal. In a patient journal, all the important information necessary for compliance and monitoring of a patient's care is kept in one place. A journal would be particularly useful in obstetrics, where compliance and self-monitoring by the patient are particularly important. However, the concept could be used in any area of care in which the health care providers are counting on the patients to not only monitor their own care but also actively participate. A journal can be a very specific educational tool for patients and their families to positively encourage participation. A portion of the journal could include a section on safety issues so that patients and their families are encouraged to be vigilant in recognizing and preventing mistakes.

In March 2002, the Joint Commission partnered with the Centers for Medicare & Medicaid Services to launch a national campaign called "Speak Up." The campaign is intended to encourage patients to become actively involved in their own health care. In response, hospitals around the United States are encouraging patients to do the following:

1. Ask questions about their own care
2. Make sure they are receiving the proper treatment
3. Educate themselves
4. Have a family or friend advocate
5. Review the credentials of any clinic, hospital, or other health care facility where care will be provided
6. Know what medications they take
7. Participate in their own health care treatment decisions

In support of this initiative, the Joint Commission provides brochures, posters, and buttons. In a 2005 survey of more than 600 Joint Commission-accredited organizations, 91 percent rated the Speak Up program as excellent, very good, or good. These health care organizations have used the resources in patient rooms, sponsoring public service announcements, Web sites, newsletters, and even staff orientation.[12]

Figure 6-1 lists some of the safety suggestions offered to patients and families on the Web site of Lowell (MA) General Hospital.[13] These types of communications are examples of health care providers pursuing active participation of patients as members of a health care team. It brings expectations more in line with reality at the same time it informs the patient about potential mistakes and irregularities that do and can exist. While this information sharing can make the patient more vigilant, the health care provider must be cognizant that such partnering needs to be done in the right way—it is important to put certain statements in the correct context. For example, while partnering with a patient to prevent wrong-site surgery, the physician and staff members should explain that wrong-site surgery occurs infrequently. In a study on the incidence of wrong-site surgery among hand surgeons, it was reported that such errors occur once in every 27,686 procedures.[14] Recently, in a study of 2,826,367 procedures from 1985 to 2004, 25 nonspine wrong-site surgeries were identified, resulting in an incidence of 1 in 112,994 surgeries.[15]

It is important to strike a balance between the art of reassurance and information sharing. Even though information sharing builds the confidence of a patient through partnering, it is essential to also consider when too much information may actually harm the patient and/or the care of the patient. Increased vigilance by the patient is important for his or her own safety, but it is also important that health care providers do not go overboard to the point where the disclosure of potential medical errors actually acts to alarm an already anxious patient. In addition, there is a point at which qualitative information becomes denuded and thus stripped of meaning, preventing a patient from focusing on the essential aspects of his or her care. Further, physicians and their staff often operate under strict time constraints, and for this reason health care providers may be unable to disclose every

Figure 6-1. Safety Information Disclosed to Patients on the Web Site of Lowell (MA) General Hospital

Your Role in Patient Safety

These are ways you can help us give you the best care:

- Speak up if you have questions or concerns about your care.

- If you don't understand something, ask! It's your body, and you have a right to know.

- Tell your doctor or nurse if something doesn't seem quite right.

- Expect health care workers to introduce themselves when they enter your room, and look for their identification badge.

- Tell the health care worker right away if you think he or she has confused you with another patient.

- Know what medicines you take and why you take them.

- Know what time of day you normally receive a medication. If it doesn't happen, ask your nurse or doctor why you didn't get your medicine.

- If you do not recognize a medication, be sure that it is for you.

- Make sure your nurse or doctor knows who you are, that is, checks your wristband or asks your name before he or she gives any medication or treatment.

- Be involved in all decisions about your treatment—you are part of the health care team.

- You might want to ask a trusted family member or friend to help you. They can help remember answers to questions and speak up for you if you cannot.

- Write down important facts your doctor tells you, so that you can look for more information later. And ask your doctor or nurse if he or she has any written information you can keep.

- Ask your doctor the purpose of any new test or medication.

- Read all medical forms and make sure you understand them before you sign anything. If you don't understand, ask your doctor or nurse to explain them.

Source: Lowell General Hospital, Lowell, Massachusetts. See the full text of the site at http://www.lowellgeneral.org/go/patients-and-vistors/for-patients/ while-you-are-here/helping-us-help-others/your-role-in-patient-safety/ your-role-in-patient-safety. Reprinted with permission.

potential risk no matter its likelihood of occurrence. These are only challenges to be faced, however, and should not be seen as obstacles.

Family-Centered Care

True patient involvement and partnering with patients can have beneficial effects on a patient's health. One particularly innovative movement is the advocacy of family-centered care. Dr. Nicholas Masi, director of family-centered care at the Joe DiMaggio Children's Hospital, Fort Lauderdale, Florida, and former practicing psychologist, is helping to create opportunities for patient and family involvement in health services.[16] In an interview with the authors, Dr. Masi explained that obstetrics was one of the first services to embrace family-centered care; however, patient demand has expanded this model of care to other services, such as pediatrics. Dr. Masi would like to see family-centered care as the norm, not only in children's health care facilities but also in adult care areas.

According to Dr. Masi, family-centered care is a different way of providing patient treatment, and effecting this change requires a cultural change in the mind-set of health care providers. At the Joe DiMaggio Children's Hospital, for example, family members are to be viewed as caregivers, not visitors; the health care practitioners are the people considered to be visitors. To support this cultural change, the organization is working on a language change to be used by staff and to be evidenced in job descriptions and other facility documents.

Positive outcomes have been particularly evident in the neonatal unit. The hospital has designed a room, somewhat like a hotel room, where parents may stay overnight to take care of their infant when discharge is imminent. This allows the parents to become comfortable with caring for their child before going home. Any issues that arise are discussed and remedied while the child is still hospitalized.

Dr. Masi is also encouraging physicians to include family members on patient rounds. He finds that when families are involved in their child's care, for example, several positive outcomes occur, including the following:

- The child's rate of return to the hospital for significant complications is reduced.
- The parent-child bond is enhanced.
- The child's risk of an incident involving social or developmental issues goes down.
- Families are better able to cope with their child's illness.

Rounds with families have been so successful in Pediatrics that the hospital system as a whole (which includes five hospitals) has hired a director of family-centered care for the adult hospitals. Rounds with families in those institutions have started with the trauma teams. Dr. Masi's organization is sponsoring even more cutting-edge family-centered initiatives, including the following:

- Family members are given a choice if they want to be involved in resuscitation.
- Family members are used as faculty in the educational process, including employee orientation. According to Dr. Masi, having a family member share his or her story is very powerful.
- Family members are sitting on committees and the board in the adult hospitals.
- Soon to be instituted, family-initiated rapid response teams will allow family members to call the rapid response team directly. The hospital has created guidelines for the family and will provide education.[17]

Informed Consent

Because an essential patient safety tool is communication, it is vital for physicians and other caregivers to establish open lines of communication with patients. Communication establishes trust and provides a framework for discussion between the caregiver and the patient that is essential to the success of information sharing. One of the first instances in which open communication is beneficial is during the informed consent process—disclosure preintervention. The informed consent process is a patient-specific form of communication, not just a document that must be completed and signed. Although the legal principles of informed consent vary from state to state, the general principles are the same:

- The proposed treatment/procedure is explained.
- The known risks and alternatives to the proposed treatment/procedure are disclosed.
- The risks of not undergoing any treatment/procedure are discussed.
- The alternatives to the proposed treatment/procedure and any associated risks are explained.

Informed consent has an ethical foundation, one in which the patient has a right to make informed decisions about his or her own body. A proper informed consent discussion and process will allow a patient to make a truly informed decision. More than this, the informed consent process is an opportunity for the patient to ask questions and receive answers. A properly executed informed consent opens dialogue and involves the patient in his or her own care. As a result, the patient feels cared for, listened to, and respected.[18] Should the patient actually incur one of the risks, he or she will have heard about it before, and there is an atmosphere that will permit open, frank communication about the patient care. Further, the patient's expectations remain in line with reality.[19] Conversely, if a patient hears for the first time about a potential complication *after* it occurs, he or she tends to become suspicious and angry.[20] It is these types of scenarios that lead a patient to become a plaintiff—or to visit a plaintiff attorney and a plaintiff attorney to take on a case. Patients want answers and want to understand what occurred, but sometimes they resort to their attorney rather than their physician. You can prevent that scenario with better communication.

One way physicians are enhancing the informed consent process and patient involvement is incorporating Web-based informed consent and educational information into this process. Harlon Wilson, president and chief executive officer of Medical Animatics, Inc., has this explanation:[21]

The use of Web-based patient education and informed consent applications provides many benefits to health care providers and patients alike. While this is still relatively new technology, the use of three-dimensional animation, graphic arts, audio narration, and interactive programming in a Web-based distance-education model is a tool that has enabled physicians to empower their patients toward understanding treatment information. The use of multimedia patient education serves three very important potential outcomes.

First, the patients become more engaged in decision making about medical treatment options and are therefore more likely to engage in the treatment process. This may include postprocedural follow-up as well as the adoption of healthier lifestyle behaviors as a result of their newly obtained knowledge.

Second, a more engaged patient is more likely to ask questions and to interact with health care providers during their follow-up visits. This opportunity for improving doctor-patient communication may impact the patients' perceptions about their physician's empathy for their medical treatment, which may go a long way toward reducing medical liability risk.

Third, physicians who use our tools have reported a 20 to 30 percent savings in chair time with patients. They are no longer drawing stick figures while providing lengthy explanations; they are instead using simplified output reports that summarize the patients' navigation and test results. Patients then require less in-depth training and have reported an improved comfort level with the legal documentation process of informed consent. The physicians' ability to focus on only the areas that need further clarification saves time and reduces medical liability risk as it relates to informed patients.

With good informed consent and patient education pre-intervention, physicians can develop good relationships with patients. A strong physician-patient relationship can reduce adversity when an error, or any adverse event, does occur. Often patients misinterpret a complication as a medical error. It may be important to define what a complication is for your patient so that if one does occur, your postintervention conversation with the patient will be much easier. At times true errors will occur, and they will need to be managed appropriately.

The informed consent process can be a valuable patient safety tool when used as a true patient education process in which medical risks as well as potential safety issues are disclosed.[22] At first, practitioners may think discussions of safety issues will lead to greater patient anxiety or mistrust of caregivers. In reality, patients want to know and want to help. It is clear that patients expect to be kept informed and involved throughout their treatment. A participant in a recent study of patient perspectives on the ideal physician commented, "I would like to be informed about what's going on. It's probably the most critical thing in having good health care. . . . Treat me like I'm human and intelligent."[23] The information provided during the informed consent process, both risks and alternatives as well as safety issues, is the type of information that could be contained in a patient journal.

Disclosing the Potential for Error

In the future, will a physician or other health care provider have an affirmative obligation to disclose potential safety issues and then be liable for failing to do so after a medical error actually comes to fruition? As more information about the incidence of medical errors comes to light, does it become a standard of care to disclose the potential for errors? At this time, it would appear unlikely that such disclosures will become standard practice. The legal analysis for such potential claims follows.

If the potential for well-known medical errors is required to be disclosed as part of the informed consent process, does a failure to disclose result in a lost opportunity for the patient to guard against the potential error? Such a claim would have to be alleged under a negligence theory and would need to be linked causally to any injury that occurred. Or is it simply that a discussion on the potential error should have been part of the informed consent process? At the present time, informed consent requirements in most jurisdictions do not embrace systemwide errors or remote risks, like wrong-site surgery.

It is probably in physicians' best interest not to confuse risks with medical errors during the informed consent discussion. As mentioned previously, you may want to define what a complication is and is not during your informed consent discussion, which may later help you in discussing any adverse event that does occur. It could help to reduce patient surprise, making postintervention disclosure less contentious. In fact, the informed consent discussion and any corresponding document can be used during postintervention discussions after an adverse outcome occurs.

Information sharing with a patient preintervention is a valuable tool that enhances a patient's health care experience. Involving patients in their own care leads to better outcomes and provides a framework for preintervention discussions. Of course, the informed consent stage is essential for disclosing the potential for material risks, but it is also a time to begin the process of involving patients more actively in their own care. Information sharing, including informed consent, helps to keep patients' expectations in line with reality. Once the provider-patient communication lines have been opened, the positive aspects of this collaboration can carry over into postintervention interactions. And it is at the postintervention point that many liability fears are realized, but those fears can—and should—be overcome.

Postintervention Communication

Full disclosure of a medical error after it has occurred has many potential advantages, including reduction of the severity and frequency of claims. Often, however, health care providers assume just the opposite—that disclosure of a medical error will result in a deterioration of the provider-patient relationship or influence the patient to seek legal action. Following are several specific concerns related to disclosure of a mistake:

- Liability implications
- Lawsuits
- Liability insurance coverage
- Reimbursement
- Peer review proceedings

A discussion of these and several related points follows.

Liability Implications

Health care organizations and physicians often fear that disclosing a medical error to the patient or family will be perceived as an admission of liability. Will the disclosure be used against the facility or the practitioner at trial? In answering this question, it is important to understand that disclosure of an error, done in the right fashion, does not mean that the facility or practitioner was negligent. There is often a misperception by the medical community as to what constitutes legal negligence.

Legal Negligence

The legal standard of negligence requires that a plaintiff prove, to a reasonable degree of medical certainty, that the conduct of a physician or other caregiver breached the applicable "standard of care" and that the breach in the care legally caused the plaintiff's injuries. As to a professional physician, the standard of care generally requires that a physician have and use the same knowledge and skill and exercise the same care as that which is usually possessed and exercised in the medical profession. A specialist must generally meet a higher standard of care: He or she must have and use the same knowledge and skill and exercise the same care as that possessed and exercised by others in the same specialty. A physician or specialist who fails to meet the applicable standard is considered negligent.

Meanwhile, a hospital or physician's practice can be held legally liable for the negligent actions of its physicians and staff (including nurses) under an agency theory as long as a causative connection to the damage is established as well. In addition, some states have extended the doctrine of corporate negligence to hospitals, finding that hospitals owe a direct duty of care to patients cared for in their facilities.

Case law in many jurisdictions establishes that an error in judgment is not negligence. A distinction is made between actual malpractice, an error in judgment, and sources of adverse outcomes that are not the fault of the physician. A mal-occurrence is not malpractice.

These legal distinctions can become blurred and, hence, a source of confusion. A physician, hospital, or other health care provider is legally negligent only when the care rendered by the physician (or hospital in the case of corporate negligence) breached the standard of care (explained above). Further, even if a health care provider has breached the standard of care, the health care provider can be liable to the plaintiff only if the plaintiff further shows that the breach in care legally caused the injuries complained of by the plaintiff (that is, generally, that the actions of the health care provider were a substantial factor in bringing about the harm incurred by the plaintiff).[24] If no such connection is made between the actions of the health care provider and the injuries incurred by the plaintiff, the health care provider is not liable for the injuries sustained by the plaintiff. In other words, as long as we are thoughtful in the way disclosure occurs, it will not be used as a judicial admission, and a plaintiff must still establish how that breach was the legal cause of the injury before liability will attach.

Statute of Limitations

Failing to disclose a medical error in a timely manner may potentially influence the statute of limitations (the period given to a potential plaintiff for filing suit). If a defendant is found to have concealed a medical error, whether actively or unintentionally, under certain circumstances such concealment may act to extend the time for filing of a professional liability lawsuit.[25]

Let us consider a situation in which a state law provides that a claimant has two years from the date of injury to file a professional liability claim and a physician has actively concealed an error in a surgery for an ulcer. Unknown to the patient, the sponge count was off, and the physician and staff were unable to locate the missing sponge. Subsequently, the patient incurred abdominal pain of unknown etiology. Five years after the ulcer surgery, during exploratory surgery in attempts to discover the source of abdominal pain, a sponge was discovered. By failing to disclose the error in sponge count, the patient had no reason to know the source of the pain could be from a retained sponge. Instead of the patient being required to file a lawsuit within two years of the first surgery, a legal principle—the "discovery rule"—could allow a plaintiff to file a lawsuit within two years of the discovery of the retained sponge, which occurred during the second surgery (five years later). Under the discovery rule, the limitation statute in malpractice cases does not start to run (i.e., the cause of action does not accrue) until the date of the discovery of the malpractice, or the date when, by the exercise of reasonable care and diligence, the patient should have discovered the wrongful act.[26]

In the above example, concealment of an error extended the statute of limitations by five years. This is a significant length of time that could have an effect on the ability to secure accurate data, records, witnesses, and recollections in defense of the malpractice action. This example, in which an error was concealed, is not to be confused with the so-called discovery rule that extends the statute of limitations when a patient, even though he or she is diligent, could have "discovered" the relationship between the care and the injury. This situation is confronted most often in misdiagnosis of cancer cases.

Research by DecisionQuest, Inc., a nationwide trial and jury consulting firm, has shown that jurors expect disclosure of medical error to occur whether it results in injury to the patient or not. This research finding is not unexpected because jurors are very much like the average patient. When asked about disclosure preferences, patients reportedly want even minor errors to be revealed to them by their physician.[27] These findings suggest that disclosure of medical mistakes may actually work in favor of the physician and the provider facility. Otherwise, jurors may perceive a cover-up and conjure up conspiracy theories and reasons that the physician or hospital is "hiding" something.

DecisionQuest advocates that the defense team consider early on how to use the communication of disclosure to its advantage. The authors have been involved in creating and implementing policies whereby disclosure has been used to effectively diffuse the patient's and family's emotions after an adverse event, resulting in a move to a fast-track claims process when appropriate. It is necessary for health care providers to be educated about such types of policies, which take time and other resources to effectively develop and in which to train health care providers.

Apologies

It has been argued that health care providers would feel more at ease in apologizing for a medical error if such apologies were prohibited from being admitted as evidence at a trial.[28] At the time of this writing, thirty-eight states have enacted sympathy/apology laws, providing immunity protections to health care providers. The content of those statutes varies, but all essentially provide some form of protection, preventing an apology or expression of empathy from being introduced as evidence of negligence in a professional liability action. It has been suggested that such laws could reduce medical errors as well as lawsuits. The real reason for this potential result is that it provides the health care provider with a perceived safe environment to apologize, one in which the apology cannot be used against a health care provider as an admission of negligence. The reality is that health care providers do not need such a law to apologize, as long as the apology is done in the right way. Doug Wojcieszak, founder and spokesperson for the Sorry Works! Coalition, agrees: "Apology laws help health care providers to get past the cultural inhibitions to disclosure that have seemingly prevented full and appropriate disclosure from taking hold in the health care industry. However, what is truly needed is education. If disclosure is done in the right way, it can be beneficial to patients, their families, and the health care providers. A law is not needed to make this happen."[29]

In the well-regarded 2002 study by Hickson and colleagues published in the *Journal of the American Medical Association*, it was discovered that nearly one-quarter of all professional liability suits (prenatal suits) were filed because a patient was angered that the health care provider had not been honest or had misled the patient.[30] Even if an apology does not prevent a lawsuit, it may at least decrease animosity and lead to a quicker resolution of the case.[31] Apologies can be useful, whether made in response to an adverse outcome or a medical error. It is important to remember that an apology can be made without an admission of fault, when appropriate, and it is important not to admit fault when no negligence exists. There will be times, however, when an admission of fault could be necessary, but you should consult legal counsel before doing so, as is discussed in more detail later in this chapter. This is another area in which training and education of health care providers and risk managers can make a real difference.

Multiple Defendants

Disclosure of a mistake can be problematic when other potential defendants may be involved with the error or complication. Consider an incident that occurs when a surgeon, an anesthesiologist, a medical specialist, and nurses are all actively involved in caring for a patient. The disclosure process must be coordinated because each provider may be a potential defendant. Questions to be addressed include, Who will speak on behalf of all involved parties at meetings with patients and/or families? What will be said and when? Each party, of course, will be wary of where blame or fault may be unintentionally placed. The logistics can become complicated but should not be an excuse for failing to disclose the facts and circumstances of an incident with the patient and/or the patient's family. As has been discussed, failure to disclose has more significant adverse effects than does disclosure to all involved. Working through the logistics and concerns is warranted and is being successfully accomplished throughout the United States.

Litigation Implications

Health care professionals fear that disclosure will prompt professional liability lawsuits, as evidenced by the fact that fear of medical malpractice litigation has been cited as the most common barrier for developing and implementing disclosure policies.[32] However, from a liability standpoint there is growing support that information sharing is an aid to the physician or hospital.

Early evidence suggests that disclosure does not result in an increase in lawsuits. For example, consider the Veterans Administration (VA) Medical Center in Lexington, Kentucky. In the 1980s, it suffered two large awards in medical malpractice cases (totaling more than $1.5 million). In 1987, the medical center adopted a disclosure policy and procedure, which involves full disclosure to the patient and/or family of a medical error that has caused injury. The disclosure includes an apology and a discussion of compensation and liability. Although the policy has resulted in some settlements where no litigation may have been instituted had the disclosure not been made, to date full disclosure has not resulted in higher liability payments.[33]

One study found that the economic benefit of disclosure is positive, resulting in reasonable settlements and fair compensation to the injured parties.[34] One of the study researchers, Steve S. Kraman, pulmonologist and hospital chief of staff at the VA Medical Center in Lexington, stated that although the total number of litigation cases increased following implementation of the full disclosure policy, the cost per case decreased dramatically.[35] On average, the medical center makes fourteen payments per year (which is a high number for a veterans hospital), but the average payment per case is only $15,000, compared with the average payment at other VA hospitals of $100,000. The cost savings here may be due largely to the lack of full-fledged litigation, which is far more expensive.

The effectiveness of the Lexington facility's disclosure policy led to implementation of a similar policy throughout all Veterans Health Administration facilities in 1995.[36] The policy requires that the medical center do the following:

- Inform the patient and/or his or her family of an event.
- Assure the patient and/or his or her family that medical measures have been implemented.
- Disclose steps that are being taken to minimize further personal or financial loss.
- Advise the patient and/or his or her family of the procedures for recovering compensation for the harm.

Can this same policy of disclosure work well in the private sector? The Veterans Health Administration system is somewhat different from a legal standpoint. Doctors working in the system are protected from personal liability and cannot be individually named in a malpractice suit. Medical malpractice lawsuits brought against a federal facility must be filed under the Federal Tort Claims Act, which bars punitive damages.[37] In addition, if a patient's injuries are military service related, he or she may qualify for financial assistance. In contrast, a physician operating in the private sector may be sued personally.[38] However, in both instances, any financial payment made on behalf of the physician must be reported to the National Practitioner's Data Bank.[39]

Despite these factors, there is no reason why similar disclosure policies implemented in the private sector would not yield the same results as those that are being seen within the Veterans Health Administration. In 2001, the University of Michigan Health System (UMHS) instituted a similar program. The health system reports that its disclosure program has saved it $2.2 million in its first year alone, and it claims that the number of lawsuits has dropped every year, from 262 in 2001 to fewer than 100 by August 2005. Further, UMHS reports that its claim reserves dropped by two-thirds and the average costs for litigation were reduced in half.[40] Other disclosure programs with variations are beginning to be adopted in organizations throughout the United States.

The substantive area of law is governed by state malpractice laws in both cases, so no legal barriers would prohibit such a system in the private sector. By implementing a system similar to that in the VA system, private sector organizations really would be implementing a risk management program that could similarly lead to reasonable settlements and just compensation to injured parties.

Although preliminary results suggest that full disclosure of medical errors can reduce liability risks, fear of the potential for litigation continues to be a significant barrier to open and honest provider-patient communication. This fear is most likely derived from the inherent nature of tort law: Its perceived intent is to punish and deter future conduct by both the wrongdoer and others who might act similarly in the future. However, this perception is not legally accurate except when punitive damages are asserted; punitive damages are claimed when a health care provider's actions are intentional or reckless.[41] This barrier to full disclosure is one that could be alleviated by the right tort reform measures. In addition, it is important that the physician or individual disclosing the medical error not discuss fault or blame to prevent the appearance of an admission of liability. Keep in mind as well that it is both the frequency and the severity of claims that health care providers are seeking to reduce.

Another barrier to full disclosure of medical errors is the fear that sharing information will lead to adverse publicity for the physician and/or the facility. Adverse publicity would affect a physician personally as well as the reputation of his or her practice, which, of course, would have a negative financial impact for the physician. For hospitals and other provider organizations, adverse publicity can lessen the community's trust and confidence in the facility and its staff members and ultimately affect market share.

Does the fear of loss of reputation make health care providers reluctant to disclose information about a medical error? In a study by Lamb and colleagues, it was found that the threat of negative news media coverage did not influence a hospital's willingness to disclose information to any of its patients.[42] In fact, proper disclosure prevents misinformation and reduces the public's perception that the hospital is hiding something. Hickson and colleagues' study of perinatal injury lawsuits further reinforces the value of open and honest communication with patients—50 percent of the lawsuits were motivated by suspicions of a cover-up.[43] If the media do request information about an adverse event, it is essential that physicians and hospitals get expert assistance from professionals in risk management and public relations and also consider patient confidentiality issues.

Liability Coverage Implications

Contracts for insurance may inadvertently inhibit disclosure reform efforts.[44] Disclosure may violate the contract of professional liability insurance between the physician and the insurance carrier and thus threaten insurance coverage for any claims related to the disclosure. Generally, physicians are prohibited by contract from hindering the defense of a claim, and some professional liability carriers require consent from the insurance carrier before the physician may apologize or admit liability. The insurance carrier may construe an apology or any other disclosure as an admission of liability, thereby violating the insurance contract, and such a violation may allow the insurance carrier to deny coverage. Done the right way, an apology or disclosure should not negatively affect coverage; however, discussions with your insurance carrier in advance are important. The same is true for professional liability coverage maintained by a hospital or other health care organization, whether coverage is for the entity itself or maintained by the entity on behalf of its employees, including physicians and nurses.

Kraman and Hamm maintain that professional liability insurers are often interested in small payouts, and for this reason insurers would have to be convinced of the economic benefit of disclosure, especially full disclosure like that implemented in the Veterans Health Administration.[45] However, this contract-related disincentive is likely to disappear as more insurance carriers become enlightened and actually encourage disclosure for obvious reasons—it reduces the potential for both frequency and severity of claims when done appropriately. More recently, enlightened professional liability insurers have begun to move to the forefront of encouraging appropriate, coordinated disclosure and should continue to educate and train accordingly. For example, one insurance program in central Pennsylvania includes an event management program that supports disclosure, when done in the right fashion. Risk management and legal professionals are available to help physicians prepare for such discussions to lessen the risk of an admission, which could be used against the physician.[46]

Peer Review Implications

Concerns specific to health care professionals involve peer review, credentialing, and licensure. Physicians and other licensed professionals may fear that disclosing a medical error would trigger peer review, sanctions, or a licensing review by a state board. For example, if a physician has documented the disclosure of several medical errors, would that situation prompt a peer review, disciplinary proceedings, or a licensing review? Such investigations would be counterproductive unless the reason for the error could truly be associated with individual competency problems.

To alleviate fears that disclosures will prompt peer review or disciplinary proceedings, it is recommended that disclosure policies and procedures make it clear that sharing information about a medical error with the patient (or patient's family) is not an admission of responsibility for purposes of peer review, sanctioning, and reporting requirements.[47] This clarification could alleviate some concerns about disclosure for physicians and other health care professionals.

Achieving Full Disclosure

The legal and cultural obstacles to full disclosure of medical errors need to be overcome so that patients (and their families) can be truly engaged as partners in the health care experience. Even though the legal concerns and fears are real, all stakeholders in this issue can have their agendas advanced by a system that embraces postintervention disclosure. The issues are complex, and the solutions will take time and investments in change. To create a culture of safety, senior leaders and management must commit to changing the status quo and convey that commitment to physicians and staff members. Many organizations start the cultural change process by developing and disseminating a policy on patient and family member communication following an error or a near miss.[48] The key issues surrounding disclosure are summarized in figure 6-2.

Disclosure Tactics

Effective patient communication needs to be incorporated into the culture of safety to promote disclosure. Recall that failed communication is often the "major instigating factor in lawsuits."[49] Patients (or their families) often file suits just to learn about the facts of what happened. Recall as well the many benefits of better provider-patient communication: a

Figure 6-2. Summary of Issues Related to Postintervention Disclosure

---

- Explain to the patient and/or family members that an unexpected error has occurred (never speculate).
- Inform them that an investigation is going to occur or has begun.
- Apologize with empathy to the patient and/or family members.
- Assure the patient and/or family members that the problem will be fixed so that the error will not occur again.
- Select the appropriate communicator.
- Involve risk management professionals.
- Assure the patient and/or family members that the patient's personal safety is of foremost importance, and describe what is being done to safeguard it.
- Do not place blame or fault.
- Provide the patient and/or family members with contact information so that they can obtain further information.
- Document the disclosure—where, when, and who was in attendance—in the patient's medical chart.
- Document specifics of the disclosure in risk management files.
- Be mindful of confidentiality implications.

---

framework for discussion, patient involvement, patients feeling like partners in their own care, improved health of the patient, and a decrease in the potential number of professional liability lawsuits. Nonetheless, postintervention communication should be accomplished with certain parameters in mind. After the occurrence of a medical error, patients want three things:

1. An explanation of what happened
2. An apology
3. An assurance that the cause will be fixed so that the error will not occur again[50]

The doctor may be the most logical communicator for disclosing an error to a patient, even when the mistake was caused by a system problem that may have been out of the physician's control. Ideally, the physician has already established an open line of communication with the patient as well as a rapport. Of course, there will be times when it is impossible for the physician to conduct the discussion or when a particular physician is just not capable of properly conducting such a discussion. For this reason, the organization should designate a properly trained backup individual. Further, even if it is the doctor communicating the error, the process should be a collaborative effort with professional risk managers and, when appropriate, legal counsel.

It is never appropriate for the physician and/or hospital to remain silent following a harmful incident, as this approach is often perceived as a cover-up by the patient or family. For documentation and verification purposes, a second individual should be in attendance during the disclosure—risk management personnel or another individual designated by the facility.

When multiple practitioners are involved, coordinate the disclosure process so that everyone's rights are protected and a unified message is delivered. The attendance of certain individuals during a discussion should always be coordinated with risk management professionals and the appropriate professional liability insurer.

The information disclosed to the patient and/or the family should be limited to what is actually known. Never speculate. In many instances, it is impossible to know immediately exactly what went wrong, but the disclosure conversation needs to take place as soon as possible after an incident, so do not wait until the investigation results are known. The patient and/or family need to be told how and/or why the incident occurred and that the cause may not be known until a later time. It is important to let the patient and family know that an investigation will be taking place and the time when further discussions may occur. The main concern should be the patient's safety and well-being. The patient must be given the information necessary for understanding how his or her continued treatment will be affected by the incident, and he or she needs to feel continued involvement in the health care experience. Disclosure is not a time to blame or place fault.

Specifically, acknowledge that an unexpected error has occurred, indicate where and when the incident took place, and share the circumstances surrounding the incident. Disclose the consequences of the error to continued treatment and who will be managing the patient's care from then on. Take time to answer questions posed by the patient and family. Be regretful if necessary, and apologize for what has occurred (not to be confused with an apology for any kind of negligent actions; in such situations you should involve legal counsel and your insurance carrier). Empathize with the patient and family and provide information on support services if necessary. Explain who has been informed of the error, the investigation and review that will take place, and steps that will be taken so the same error will not happen in the future. Let the patient and family know that as more information becomes available, they will be informed. In the meantime, provide them with contact information so that any questions that arise in the future can be answered.

Involve risk management personnel as well as liability insurers from an informational point of view. Risk management professionals can provide valuable insight into disclosure practices and assist in coordinating messages. Document the disclosure and any subsequent conversations in your investigative peer review file. In the patient's medical records, it should only be noted that a conversation took place and when, where, and who was in attendance. All further details, including what was discussed, that the family and/or patient had the opportunity to ask questions, and that assistance was offered, should be documented in risk management files. Failure to document the disclosure may lead jurors to believe that the conversation never took place. In addition, some states require mandatory disclosure of certain medical errors. In such cases, a letter such as the one shown in figure 6-3 must be sent to the patient.

There are rare circumstances when it may be necessary to withhold information from a patient and/or family. On occasion, the potential harm to a patient's health will outweigh the benefit of disclosure, or there may even be psychological reasons for withholding information. In these instances, document the

Figure 6-3.   Sample Letter to Patient for Medical Error Disclosure Documentation

Date: _____

Dear _____,

ABC Hospital is committed to providing quality medical care for its patients and the communities it serves. Despite constant and committed efforts to provide and improve patient care, medical complications sometimes unfortunately occur.

ABC Hospital is committed to respecting the rights of patients and their families to be informed about the occurrence of serious events, and to analyze such events to improve patient care and prevent recurrence of such events. This notification confirms our discussion with you concerning the occurrence of a serious event and the steps that [we are taking] [were taken] to remedy the problem.

On [date of notification] at [time of notification], a meeting was held with [names of those in attendance].

As we discussed, [details of the event].

We strongly encourage you to call [name of risk manager or patient safety officer] at [phone number] if any further questions or concerns arise. Your continued satisfaction with the care [you/your family member] receive[s] at ABC Hospital is our primary goal, and we would appreciate any other questions or comments that you may have regarding this matter.

_____

[Printed name of staff who provided notification]

_____

[Signature of staff who provided notification]

Note: This example meets the requirements of some state laws for the disclosure of medical errors to patients. Consult legal counsel for the requirements for such disclosure in your jurisdiction.

Source: James W. Saxton, Esquire, Stevens & Lee, Lancaster, Pennsylvania.

reasons for withholding the information. Put generic information regarding the circumstances in the patient's chart, but set forth the specific reasons for withholding information in the risk management file.

Of course, if it is suspected that a patient's death was caused by a medical error, it makes this process even more important. It is necessary for the process of disclosure in such a situation to be handled in a timely manner.

Once the disclosure process has been initiated, what is most important is that caregivers learn from the error. Although there is often a desire to quickly move beyond an unpleasant situation, it is critical to conduct a complete analysis of what happened and why. In other words, there are two important obligations when a medical error occurs. First, by properly sharing information about the incident with the patient and/or family, health care professionals will have met their ethical and, at times, legal responsibilities. Full disclosure will reduce the risk of liability claims and minimize the potential for a large and severe judgment award. Second, full disclosure sets the stage for performance improvement by bringing together those involved so that preventive measures can be taken. In essence, the health care providers now possess information on how and why certain medical errors occur, which provide the means for future prevention.

Disclosure and Confidentiality

A component of the provider-patient relationship is confidentiality. Physicians and other health care professionals are generally prohibited from disclosing a patient's medical information to others without the patient's consent,[51] which could prevent the disclosure of medical errors to the patient's family. Privacy regulations promulgated by the U.S. Department of Health and Human Services (which are amendments to the Health Insurance Portability and Accountability Act) implicate the disclosure of medical information (and potentially medical errors) to a patient's "family member, other relative, or a close personal friend of the [patient], or any other person identified by the [patient]."[52] The health care provider, however, is permitted to do so only with the consent of the patient; where the patient has had an opportunity to object but has failed to do so; or where, based on the exercise of the health care provider's professional judgment, he or she reasonably can infer that the patient does not object to disclosure.[53] If, however, the patient is not present or has not had the opportunity to agree or to object to disclosure because of incapacity or an emergency, the health care provider may disclose information that is directly relevant to the individual's involvement with the patient's care if, under the health care provider's professional judgment, the provider believes that the disclosure is in the best interest of the patient.

These regulations are a legal concern that health care providers need to be aware of and follow where appropriate. In addition, health care providers should be aware that these regulations specifically provide that if a state statute allows more stringent privacy requirements, then the state law is applicable and needs to be followed.[54] For this reason, health care providers covered by the regulations must understand their particular state's laws regarding confidentiality and privacy of medical information.

Legal Risks versus Patient Safety

When communicated in the right way by the right people at the right time, information sharing and disclosure are beneficial to all participants—the patient and health care providers. For the patient, it can lead to better health outcomes. The fears of health care providers about information sharing and disclosure are understandable but need to be overcome, which can be accomplished without increasing professional liability exposure when the right approach is taken. The development of effective policies and the education of health care providers and risk managers are essential to alleviate their fears of the effect of information sharing and disclosure on health care providers' liability, insurance coverage, reimbursement, peer review, credentialing, and licensing. Effective information sharing and disclosure, in fact, can result in a reduction of both the frequency and severity of claims.

Effective preintervention communication establishes a discussion framework that has many benefits, including improved patient-practitioner partnerships and better patient care and outcomes. State laws generally require that a patient be informed of a proposed medical treatment or procedure as well as its risks and alternatives and the risks of not undergoing the treatment or procedure. This process allows a patient to make a truly informed decision and, when done properly, keeps a patient's expectations in line with reality. Preintervention communication is also an opportunity to solidify the patient-practitioner partnership.

Patient partnering is an important aspect of promoting a culture of safety. It allows a patient to be truly involved in his or her own care, which strengthens the caregiver-patient bond and promotes the health of the patient. This in turn can lead to a decrease in the incidence of medical errors and resulting professional liability claims.

If a medical mistake does occur, health care providers face many obstacles that can (but should not) prevent the sharing of information with a patient. These obstacles include liability implications, litigation implications, reputation issues, liability coverage, and peer review ramifications. Even though all of these impediments are real, they are often overstated. Postintervention disclosure done in the right way, as noted previously, can actually lead to a decrease in professional liability lawsuits, because the patient and the family are informed and involved, and confusion and anger are diffused. Further, open disclosure of incidents allows health care professionals to learn from medical errors so that similar occurrences can be prevented in the future. As the VA hospital in Kentucky has found, open and honest communication can lead to a decrease in liability claim payouts and lawsuits.

Being aware of the potential legal, cultural, and regulatory issues in information sharing will promote more effective information sharing and patient involvement. True patient involvement can promote the culture of safety for patients that everyone is looking to achieve. It is time to move the sharing of information with patients to the next level. Although at first it seems counterintuitive, a more informed and educated patient is a safer patient and one whose expectations are more realistic. Many of the perceived legal barriers to pre- and postintervention disclosure can be overcome through education and initiative.

References

1. B. A. Liang, "A System of Medical Error Disclosure," *Quality and Safety in Health Care* 11 (March 2002): 64–68.
2. G. B. Hickson, C. F. Federspiel, J. W. Pichert, C. S. Miller, J. Gauld-Jaeger, and P. Bost, "Patient Complaints and Malpractice Risk," *Journal of the American Medical Association* 287, no. 22 (2002): 2951–57; M. B. Kapp, "Legal Anxieties and Medical Mistakes," *Journal of General Internal Medicine* 12, no. 12 (1997): 787–88.
3. W. Levinson, D. L. Roter, J. P. Mullooly, V. T. Dull, and R. M. Frankel, "Physician-Patient Communication: The Relationship with Malpractice Claims among Primary Care Physicians and Surgeons," *Journal of the American Medical Association* 227, no. 7 (1997): 553–59.
4. J. B. Sexton, E. J. Thomas, and R. L. Helmreich, "Error, Stress, and Teamwork in Medicine and Aviation: Cross Sectional Surveys," *British Medical Journal* 320 (March 2000): 745–49.
5. T. H. Gallagher, A. D. Waterman, A. G. Ebers, V. J. Fraser, and W. Levinson, "Patients' and Physicians' Attitudes Regarding the Disclosure of Medical Errors," *Journal of the American Medical Association* 289, no. 8 (2003): 1001–7.
6. M. Ringel, "Mistakes in Medicine," Nexus (March/April 2003) [http://www.nexuspub.com/articles/2003/march2003/zen_mar_2003.htm].
7. B. A. Liang, "Error in Medicine: Legal Impediments to U.S. Reform," *Journal of Health Politics, Policy and Law* 24, no. 1 (1999): 27–58.
8. L. T. Kohn, J. M. Corrigan, and M. S. Donaldson, eds., *To Err Is Human: Building a Safer Health System* (Washington, DC: National Academies Press, 1999).
9. See G. B. Hickson, E. W. Clayton, P. B. Githens, and F. A. Sloan, "Factors that Prompted Families to File Medical Malpractice Claims Following Perinatal Injuries," *Journal of the American*

Medical Association 267 (1992): 1359–63; C. Vincent, M. Young, and A. Phillips, "Why Do People Sue Doctors? A Study of Patients and Relatives Taking Legal Action," *Lancet* 343 (1994): 1609–13; S. S. Kraman and G. Hamm, "Risk Management: Extreme Honesty May Be the Best Policy," *Annals of Internal Medicine* 131, no. 12 (1999): 963–67.

10. Levinson et al., "Physician-Patient Communication: The Relationship with Malpractice Claims Among Primary Care Physicians and Surgeons."

11. Liang, "A System of Medical Error Disclosure."

12. See http://www.jointcommission.org/GeneralPublic/Speak+Up/about_speakup.htm, accessed October 4, 2007.

13. Web site of Lowell General Hospital: http://www.lowellgeneral.org.

14. E. G. Meinberg and P. J. Stern, "Incidence of Wrong-Site Surgery among Hand Surgeons," *Journal of Bone & Joint Surgery* 85, no. 2 (2003): 193–97.

15. M. R. Kwaan, D. M. Studdert, M. J. Zinner, and A. A. Gawande, "Incidence, Patterns, and Prevention of Wrong-Site Surgery," *Archives of Surgery* 141 (April 2006): 353–58.

16. Author interview with Nicholas Masi, MD, director of family-centered care at the Joe DiMaggio Children's Hospital, Fort Lauderdale, Florida, May 2, 2003.

17. Conference call with Nicholas Masi, MD, and Maggie M. Finkelstein, Esq., October 5, 2007.

18. T. L. Leaman and J. W. Saxton, *Preventing Malpractice: The Co-active Solution* (New York: Plenum Publishing Co., 1993).

19. T. L. Leaman and J. W. Saxton, *Managed Care Success: Reducing Risk while Increasing Patient Satisfaction* (Frederick, MD: Aspen Publishers, Inc., 1998), 195.

20. Ibid.

21. Correspondence with Harlon Wilson, president and chief executive officer of Medical Animatics, October 5 2007.

22. Leaman and Saxton, *Managed Care Success: Reducing Risk while Increasing Patient Satisfaction*, 201.

23. D. S. Main, C. Tressler, A. Staudenmaier, K. A. Nearing, J. M. Westfall, and M. Silverstein, "Patient Perspectives on the Doctor of the Future," *Family Medicine* 34, no. 4 (2002): 251–57.

24. M. B. Kapp, "Medical Error versus Malpractice," *DePaul Journal of Health Care Liability* 1 (Summer 1997): 751, 752; see also L. Gostin, "A Public Health Approach to Reducing Error: Medical Malpractice as a Barrier," *Journal of the American Medical Association* 283, no. 13 (2000): 1742–43.

25. Kapp, "Legal Anxieties and Medical Mistakes."

26. B. A. Gardner and H. C. Black, eds., *Black's Law Dictionary*, 6th ed. (St. Paul, MN: West Publishing Co., 1991), 466.

27. A. B. Witman, D. M. Park, and S. B. Hardin, "How Do Patients Want Physicians to Handle Mistakes? A Survey of Internal Medicine Patients in an Academic Setting," *Archives of Internal Medicine* 156 (December 1996): 2565–69.

28. A. W. Wu, "Handling Hospital Errors: Is Disclosure the Best Defense?" *Annals of Internal Medicine* 131 (December 1999): 970–72.

29. Author interview with Doug Wojcieszak, founder and spokesperson, the Sorry Works! Coalition, October 4, 2007.

30. Hickson et al., "Patient Complaints and Malpractice Risk"; see also M. B. Kapp, "Legal Anxieties and Medical Mistakes."

31. L. O. Prager, "New Laws Let Doctors Say 'I'm Sorry' for Medical Mistakes," *American Medical News* 43, no. 31 (2000): 8.

32. R. M. Lamb, D. M. Studdert, R. M. Bohmer, D. M. Berwick, and T. A. Brennan, "Hospital Disclosure Practices: Results of a National Survey," *Health Affairs* 22, no. 2 (2003): 73–83.

33. Ibid.

34. Kraman and Hamm, "Risk Management: Extreme Honesty May Be the Best Policy."

35. Ibid.

36. Veterans Health Administration, *Patient Safety Improvement* (Washington, DC: Department of Veterans Affairs, 1988), 1051/1.

37. 28 U.S.C. § 2674.

38. 42 U.S.C. §§ 11101 et seq. (Health Care Quality Improvement Act of 1986).

39. Kraman and Hamm, "Risk Management: Extreme Honesty May Be the Best Policy."

40. M. Glabman, "Will 'Mea Culpa' Work for Health Plans Too?" *Managed Care Magazine*, January 2007 [http://www.managedcaremag.com/archives/0701/0701.apology.html]. Accessed October 2, 2007.

41. See State Farm Mutual Automobile Ins. Co. v. Campbell, 538 U.S. __, 123 S. Ct. 1513; 155 L. Ed. 2d 585 (2003).

42. Lamb et al., "Hospital Disclosure Practices: Results of a National Survey."

43. Hickson et al., "Patient Complaints and Malpractice Risk."

44. Liang, "Error in Medicine: Legal Impediments to U.S. Reform."

45. Kraman and Hamm, "Risk Management: Extreme Honesty May Be the Best Policy."

46. Central Pennsylvania Physicians Risk Retention Group insurance program includes a risk management program for all insureds. See http://cpprrg.com, accessed January 2008.

47. American Society for Healthcare Risk Management, *Perspective on Disclosure of Unanticipated Outcome Information* (Chicago: ASHRM, 2001).

48. Ibid.
49. Leaman and Saxton, *Managed Care Success*, 133; see also Wu, "Handling Hospital Errors."
50. C. Johnson and S. Horton, "Owning Up to Errors; Put an End to the Blame Game," *Nursing* 31, no. 6 (2001): 54.
51. 45 C.F.R. §§ 160 & 164.
52. 45 C.F.R. § 164.510(b)(1)(i).
53. 45 C.F.R. § 164.510(b)(2)(i)–(iii).
54. 45 C.F.R. § 160.202.

7

Patient Involvement in System Failure Analysis: Engaging the Overlooked Partner

Theresa M. Zimmerman and Geraldine Amori

"All that I wanted to do was help resolve the problem, not sue the hospital."

Samantha, a pleasant-looking older woman, sat at her breakfast table sharing her story. After receiving the diagnosis of breast cancer, Samantha underwent surgery, chemotherapy, and radiation. During the course of treatment, her surgical site became bright red, hot, and swollen. "I could feel a lump and it was growing. I kept being told by caregivers that it was normal and not to be concerned."

Samantha knew something wasn't right and scheduled an appointment with her physician. While the office nurse was palpating the swollen area, it ruptured and drained all over Samantha. The nurse grabbed the nearest trash can, held it up to the wound until it was done draining, and left to get the doctor. Samantha described the event as one of the most humiliating of her life. Chemotherapy and radiation therapy could not continue until the infection was treated, the wound filled and healed. It took months of additional time with the unknown impact of delayed cancer therapy.

Following this episode, Samantha sought information from the hospital and her surgeon. She wanted to know what had caused the infection. Both parties pointed their fingers at the other as the cause. The infection would later be labeled a hospital-acquired infection.

Samantha began asking more questions. She wanted to know how something like this could happen, how often patients get this type of infection, and if the hospital and physicians were doing something to prevent such infections. She never received satisfactory answers to her questions, so she sought the help of the state legislature. Samantha testified before committees and asked that hospitals publicly report hospital-acquired wound infection rates. Her efforts received much press attention.[1]

Unfortunately, events like those depicted in the story above are not uncommon. Patients such as Samantha, and their family members, often don't get their questions answered and are frustrated by barriers that prevent open sharing of information. Samantha did not sue her providers. Instead, she sought help from an outside resource, her state legislature. Samantha was later asked if her involvement in a root cause analysis of the event would have made a difference. She responded by saying that if she had been assured that the hospital and surgeon were working together to really address the problem, she would have been satisfied and would not have sought further assistance.

A Historical Perspective

The provision of health care has historically been perceived as magical, mystical, and a sovereign domain of professionals.[2] Healing the sick involved special knowledge and skill revered by communities. The physician reigned supreme, and the system supported the power of his professional sovereignty.[3] Although today we may laugh at that archaic notion and even eschew admitting it still exists today at some level, the premise behind that primitive belief is not completely unwarranted.

Time pressures and bureaucratic responses to the business of medicine have further caused practitioners to detach psychologically and emotionally from the object of our actions—our patients.[4] As practitioners become more detached from patients and their families, some key aspects of health care are being abandoned:

- The patient and family are no longer the determinants of appropriate care.
- Human interaction and trust are no longer an essential element of the relationship.
- Providers who feel they don't have enough time are no longer psychologically available to patients.
- Treating the whole person is no longer the goal; symptom management can become the focus.

Movements have long existed to engage patients and families in the health care experience. Organizations such as the Institute for Family-Centered Care (www.familycenteredcare .org) and the Picker Institute (www.pickerinstitute.org) were created to support and guide institutions in their engagement efforts. Nonetheless, initiatives have been spotty, and the liability fears associated with increased transparency have had a limiting effect.

The most progressive work is being done in oncology and pediatric care, where patients' and families' relationships with physicians span a longer period of time. Caregivers and consumers in these environments have more opportunity to create meaningful partnership interactions. Some health care organizations involve patients in very limited ways, such as soliciting input about how to arrange the physical environment. Greater engagement of patients and families in the daily clinical operations of the organization is often restricted due to legal concerns.

The Role of Patients in the System

What is the role of the patient in the health care system? At the very heart of this question is the role of health care in society. Historically, we've thought of medicine as existing to meet the needs of patients. With the emergence of new technologies, the advent of insurance, and other external influences, medicine has by necessity become a business. For this business to survive, it needs to generate income, which means the focus is often on the bottom line.

Patient-Focused versus Patient-Centered Care

If health care truly existed for those it serves—patients and families—then the focus would, by definition, be on meeting the psychological and physical needs of patients and families. The disparate goals of maintaining business viability and satisfying patient and family requirements create a dynamic tension. This tension is often at the heart of the struggle about how transparent a health care organization is willing to be in those areas where it is financially or legally vulnerable.

Some organizations have committed to patient-focused care. However, this type of care is different from patient-centered care. In a patient-focused environment, those who deliver the care retain control. Care decisions are made by providers and delivered to patients. Often the patient is seen as a passive recipient of system successes and failures. Rarely is the patient's perspective or input sought on how health care is being delivered or how it is being evaluated and improved.

By contrast, a patient-centered approach supports the assertion that patients are the determinants of appropriate care. In this approach, the patient is an integral part of every aspect and concern of care delivery.[5] Here, the patient's needs drive the system, whereas in patient-focused care, the provider's needs drive the system. In patient-centered care, patients are both participants and integral elements in the system, and they are equal partners with providers.

Trust and Transparency

The study by Blendon and colleagues published in the *New England Journal of Medicine* in 2002[6] demonstrated the chasm of trust that has developed between those who deliver health care and those who receive it. In this study, most physicians

(86 percent) reportedly believed that hospital reports of errors should be kept confidential to encourage open discussion among colleagues. A majority of laypersons (62 percent) favored public reporting of errors.

At the heart of this trust chasm is the consumer's belief that the health care system will neither police nor improve itself without public accountability. This belief is further evident in the fact that jury decisions are often influenced by the conviction that there is collusion among those in the health care industry.[7] The implication of these attitudes is that health care professionals have come to fear the very people they serve.

Illustrating this shift in the patient-practitioner relationship are comments from a physician's wife who was overheard by one of the authors to say, "I just called my husband at his office. He couldn't talk. He said there were 30 potential plaintiffs in his waiting room."

Patient-centered care and transparency can help rebuild the public's trust in health care and mend potentially adversarial relationships between patients and providers. Consider how different the introductory scenario for this chapter would have been if Samantha had participated with her caregivers in an investigation of the cause of her surgical wound infection. She would have gotten her questions answered and would have known that her concerns were being taken seriously by the providers. Samantha would have also learned that the cause of an infection is not always certain but that physicians and hospital staff are doing what they can to prevent this complication. Samantha's trust in the health care system might have been restored.

Involving Patients in Systems Failure Analysis

Systems failure analysis (SFA) refers to any evaluation of health care processes conducted for the purpose of improving patient safety. This includes root cause analysis, proactive risk assessment (such as failure mode and effects analysis), and other forms of system safety evaluation. Patients and family members are part of the system of health care, and as such, they have a stake in creating safer systems. Their contribution during an SFA offers an invaluable perspective that is often not apparent to those working within the systems of care. (Throughout this section, the term *patient* refers to both patients themselves and their family members.)

Benefits of Patient Involvement

When caregivers commit to embracing patients as partners, inclusion of their point of view during an SFA is a logical extension of this partnership. The patient's perspective of the course of health care events as well as what they observe to be problems are an essential contribution to the evaluation. Without patient input, it is impossible to fully evaluate the entire gamut of system failures.

A secondary benefit of patient involvement is rebuilding of trust. The patient recognizes the organization takes both actual and potential errors seriously and is striving to enhance the reliability of the system.

A third, and less obvious, benefit is to reassure the patient that his or her input is valued as a respected participant in care.

Providers also benefit from patient involvement. Unless there is litigation, it is rare for caregivers to find out what patients see or hear during the care process. Even in those rare situations where patients share their experience with providers, it is usually in the context of a complaint that needs to be resolved. In those circumstances, the provider is usually looking for things to say or do to resolve the issue or make the patient feel better. Almost never is there an opportunity to simply hear what was experienced by the patient.

Patient participation in an SFA can range from simply sharing their observations to participation in the entire evaluation process. In either case, the results of the SFA, including efforts to modify the system and the outcome of those modifications, should be communicated to the patient participant. Such openness validates the value of the patient's involvement and affirms that promises made to improve patient safety are being kept.

Including the patient as part of the SFA team is laudable; however, logistics can be troublesome. How do we ensure that organization and practitioner legal rights are not diminished or violated? What can be done to manage liability risks while enhancing everyone's participation and learning? What role can the patient play? How can we ensure that emotional harm already inflicted is not exacerbated by patient participation in the evaluation process? How can we prevent other injured parties (providers and staff) from being berated by the patient participant? How can we stop patient participation from having a chilling effect on open and honest discussions by caregivers at meetings? While there are no clear-cut answers to these questions, these perceived barriers are not as difficult to overcome as one might think.

Risk and Liability Considerations

Expanding the patients' role in their own care, especially when that care has resulted in an injury, naturally creates legal concerns for organizations and practitioners. The potential for greater liability exposure creates barriers that may not be easily overcome. While a patient's participation in the SFA process allows for introduction of a valuable and unique perspective, it does interject an "outsider" into a process typically granted discovery protections under law. There is some legitimacy to these liability concerns; however, by systematically addressing these fears, it is possible for health care teams to successfully partner with patients during an SFA.

Practitioners often fear transparency, citing the possibility of increased litigation. Yet failure to provide sufficient information to patients in an open, forthcoming manner is the basis for much of the litigation we seek to avoid.[8] In 2001, the Joint Commission first announced the standard of disclosure of unanticipated events as a responsibility inherent to patient trust.[9] Almost immediately health care organizations expressed overwhelming concern that the number of lawsuits filed against them would exponentially increase.[10] Nonetheless, organizations such as the University of Michigan Health System, the Veterans Administration Hospital in Lexington, Kentucky, and others are experiencing a reduction in litigation costs as a direct benefit of a well-run disclosure process.[11] As with disclosure, the suggestion that patients should be involved in SFAs will likely raise legal and confidentiality concerns for some organizations. Yet given the positive monetary and psychological impact of properly managed disclosure, it is logical to conclude that positive economic and psychological benefits may arise from involving patients in SFAs.

Legal Concerns

Patients and providers may both have legal concerns prior to participating in the SFA process. Patients may want to include their lawyers in the meeting or fear that they are "signing away" their rights to litigate. Caregivers may feel that what is discussed during the meeting will be used against them should a lawsuit occur. To address these concerns, one must first recognize that the SFA process is not a legal proceeding and should not be treated as such. The comments of the SFA participants are used solely for the purpose of information gathering and quality improvement. The SFA must be treated as separate and distinct from the risk management process of early resolution or preparation for potential future litigation. Furthermore, participants in the SFA process must understand these distinctions beforehand so that patient involvement is perceived as being safe and beneficial to all parties.

The question of having lawyers in the room during an SFA is broader than the issue of patient participation. The goal of the SFA process is to identify latent and root causes that have contributed, or may contribute in the future, to an adverse event or a near miss. Any individual who is present during the process can potentially inhibit open and honest communication among the SFA team members. Individuals who may compromise the integrity of the evaluation process should be excluded from the discussions or be afforded only limited participation. In some system analyses, patient involvement throughout the entire process could be intimidating to health care providers. Inviting a lawyer (who has a defense or plaintiff's agenda as the main reason for attending) to join the SFA team could be the death knell of a potentially successful investigation. Don't make hard and fast rules without weighing the risks and benefits. What is most important is consistency. For example, don't invite lawyers to attend SFA meetings *only* when a patient will be in the room.

Confidentiality Issues

Whether the SFA information will become discoverable once outsiders are invited to participate is another legal concern that must be considered on a facility-by-facility basis. State and/or federal privileges may exist to protect the confidentiality of quality and performance improvement activities. However, those protections may be waived if the organization's policies are strict in not allowing outside participants to sit on quality improvement committees. To retain confidentiality protections, the organization's policies governing such committees (including SFA teams) should allow for attendance of ad hoc members for purposes of information gathering and sharing. Review your sentinel event, root cause analysis, quality/performance improvement, and other related policies to be sure that ad hoc members, including patients, are allowed to participate in discussions.

Hospital medical staff bylaws should also be reviewed and edited to ensure that the medical staff clearly support patient participation in SFAs. Hospital and medical staff policy statements that allow for people outside of the organization to attend meetings conducted for quality and performance improvement purposes should assist in preserving the integrity of the SFA process.

Because each state has differing quality and peer review protections, legal counsel should explore possible state-specific complications that might stem from sharing confidential communications, information, and evidence with potential litigants (patients and other third parties). Additionally, have legal counsel review existing state and federal legislation, regulations, and case law to determine how best to word organizational and medical staff policies related to patient involvement in SFAs.

Once the organization has crafted properly worded policies, it remains imperative that it conducts SFAs with a high level of confidentiality and under stringent guidelines to protect the integrity of the process. All participants should be cautioned not to take written information from the room, electronically record discussions or take pictures, or talk about the proceedings of the meeting or any related matter post-adjournment. At the beginning of the meeting, explain its purpose and cite the statutory or regulatory language that affords quality and peer review protections to the meeting discussions.

Organizations may question whether the patient should sign a confidentiality agreement prior to participating in the SFA. This suggestion flies in the face of the public demand for openness and transparency. Although it may be reasonable and legal to request such documents, it does not support the patient-centered approach that is being advocated here.

Identifying and Preparing SFA Participants

Although many individuals bring their observations into the room during the SFA, there are essentially three key perspectives: those of the organization, the patient, and the caregiver. The needs and expectations of stakeholders representing each of these perspectives must be addressed before bringing everyone together.

An adverse medical event is psychologically traumatic for everyone involved—the physician, nurses and other caregivers, the patient, and the organization's leaders. For this reason, all parties must be carefully screened and prepared prior to the

SFA meeting. Particular care must be taken in selecting the patient or family who may participate, as involvement in the SFA could do even more harm by exposing them to the event again[12] as well as eliciting a potentially negative reception from the health care team. To minimize the possibility of a nonproductive or destructive encounter within the SFA process, it is essential that:

- The psychological readiness and appropriateness of participants from the three key stakeholder groups are seriously considered
- Due care is taken in preparing all participants for the encounter
- Management and debriefing of the meeting are handled respectfully and thoroughly
- Participants receive some type of follow-up communication after the meeting

Recommendations for managing these factors for the key stakeholder groups are described in the next section.

Stakeholder: The Organization

Not every organization is ready to embrace patient participation in the SFA process. The business imperative of transparency has only recently began to take hold in health care organizations,[13] and safety improvement strategies that incorporate a patient-centered philosophy have yet to gain widespread acceptance. It may not be advisable to involve patients in the SFA process if "red flag" situations such as the following exist:

- The facility and its providers (or the specific caregivers involved in the event) have an adversarial relationship. In this circumstance, the SFA meeting could become a forum for accusation and finger-pointing between the entities. This could cause serious psychological damage to all participants.

- Employees involved in adverse events are often subjected to punitive discipline. In this environment, employees often become defensive. Fear of not being supported by the organization can have a chilling effect on participants' willingness to openly consider the patient's perspective.

Even in organizations where such red flag situations exist, there are often individuals in positions of leadership who are willing to give patient involvement a chance. These individuals are vital to guiding the organization through the uncertainty that accompanies transparency and a patient-centered approach. Furthermore, one success will generate even more successes. The organization that discovers patient participation in an SFA is worthwhile is more likely to consider involving patients in the future.

Organizations willing to consider patient participation in an SFA should establish a screening process that is conducted prior to each analysis. Although this may seem redundant, remember that each adverse event elicits different organizational concerns and vulnerabilities. Situations that may raise considerable angst are events involving high-profile community members, significant adverse outcomes for a baby or child, errors made by hospital employees, or situations in which the actions were of such an egregious nature that culpability is almost certain. These situations may require extra care and careful management of the patient participation process.

Screen for Readiness

Responsibility for managing the SFA often falls to the patient safety or quality/risk management department. While individuals from any of these departments could assess organizational readiness for patient participation, it is probably best done by the risk manager. Frequently this individual is skilled in engaging patients while maintaining awareness of the psychological and legal implications of all interactions. If your organization's risk manager lacks these skills, seek assistance from patient advocacy, social services, or the organization's ethicist. What you want is an objective evaluation of your organization's readiness for open dialogue and transparency in the SFA process.

Prepare the Organization

When it's clear the organization is ready to commit to the patient involvement in an SFA, key leaders within the organization must be educated about the process, the expectations, and the possible variety of outcomes. Key leaders who should be educated include the chief medical officer, the chief nursing officer, and any other senior leaders who are championing the cause of patient involvement. At a minimum, these individuals should understand that:

- The goal of patient participation in the SFA is to discover system failures that might become evident as the patient shares what he or she observed.
- Patients and caregivers will be screened and prepared ahead of the meeting to ensure open, nonadversarial interactions.
- Guidelines will be established to protect the SFA proceedings from inappropriate internal and external disclosure.
- Patients and caregivers will be provided support after the meeting to manage any emotional ramifications stemming from the process.

It is essential that individuals in key leadership positions pledge to support the notion of patient involvement. Otherwise, that support may dwindle if caregivers begin to express concerns about having a patient in the room during an SFA. Leadership must be committed and willing to take the risk and provide support for providers and caregivers who may view themselves as vulnerable to retaliation. Providers and caregivers must feel safe from unwarranted disciplinary actions that could result from information divulged during the SFA process.

Stakeholder: The Patient

It is a given that patients and/or family members who are invited to participate in the SFA will have psychological concerns. Following an adverse event, their relationship with the health care system is in a state of vulnerable trust. Their prior beliefs about the system and caregivers' ability to heal have been jeopardized. Fears about retribution for pointing out errors and system failure are greatest in those situations where the patient has a need for further care.

The health care environment is unfamiliar to most patients. They may be reluctant to offer improvement recommendations, or they may do just the opposite—offer lots of suggestions that originate from other more familiar settings. In either situation, the disparity of experience and knowledge between the patient and the health care members of the SFA team can precipitate divisive partisanship if not properly addressed prior to and during the meeting. The facilitator of the SFA process must be prepared to skillfully avert nonverbal divisiveness, verbal defensiveness, and other destructive behavior that may be exhibited by the patient and caregiver participants.

Screen for Readiness

Screening patients for participation in an SFA should not be a separate, formal process from the usual provider-patient discussion that occurs after an event. Avoid a formal, separate assessment, as it can set up an expectation of participation that might later be withdrawn because the patient is not a good candidate. The emotional impact of reviewing the details of care to determine the causes of adverse outcomes may outweigh the benefit of family participation in the SFA.[14]

Rarely should family members of a deceased patient be considered for participation in the SFA. The analysis happens very soon after the event, and the family is often too busy managing funeral details as well as dealing with acute grief. Examining the care that may have contributed to the patient's death could exacerbate normal grieving processes. The same may be true in situations where the patient was significantly harmed and requires substantial ongoing care. The family's mental and emotional energy is often focused on the care of their loved one, and the SFA discussion could exacerbate their already heightened awareness of the patient's vulnerability and the potential for additional imminent errors.

In those situations where the patient (or family member) may be psychologically capable, emotionally ready, intellectually able, and attitudinally appropriate, the question of participation can be broached. Do this during a follow-up conversation, not at the time of the initial error disclosure. Whoever approaches the patient to participate in the SFA should be sensitive to his or her current emotional state. If the primary emotion being expressed by the patient is anger or a desire to litigate, this may not be a good candidate for participation. Assessing the patient's emotional suitability requires an understanding of human nature, culturally defined responses to emotional trauma, and cultural beliefs about health care.

The potential patient SFA participant should also be evaluated to determine if he or she understands what is being asked of them and if he or she is able to do it without becoming confused. Most importantly, it is essential the patient recognize that he or she would bring information of value to the SFA and a crucial perspective to the process.

Be sure to ascertain whether a patient desires solely to punish caregivers for an error or if their primary goal is to ensure that the error and resultant injury are not repeated. The patient should also exhibit sufficient emotional and intellectual readiness to handle the SFA process, including meeting with the caregivers who were personally involved in the event.

In 2004, Exempla Lutheran Medical Center in Wheat Ridge, Colorado, invited the father of a child who experienced an adverse event to participate in the root cause analysis. According to David Munch, MD, chief clinical and quality officer at Exempla, the decisive factors for including the father in the SFA process included:[15]

- He was never critical of people and even praised many caregivers for their efforts.
- He focused his concerns on our broken processes, poor communication, and our inability to involve the family in the child's care even though they were quite familiar with her condition.
- His daughter fully recovered from the event, although her care was not ideal.
- He had a sophisticated understanding of organizational dynamics and knew that solutions would only be achieved through systems improvement, not individual blame.

A decision tree to assist in judging patient/family readiness for involvement in an SFA and suggested actions is provided in figure 7-1.

Prepare the Patient

The well-being of the patient (or family member) who will be involved in an SFA must be a primary concern. The patient must be adequately prepared for the experience and supported during and after the analysis sessions conclude. It is crucial to keep the lines of communication open and make patients aware of the positive changes that were instituted after the event and ongoing performance monitoring. Patient preparation must include sharing information about all of the elements listed in figure 7-2.

Stakeholder: The Caregivers

The most diverse group of SFA participants are the caregivers who will be involved in the analysis. Physicians, nurses, and other caregivers have learned to rely on the risk manager for guidance through potential litigious situations; however, when patient participation in the SFA is suggested, caregivers may express distrust and fear. Physicians, and occasionally nurses or other professionals, have personal liability insurance, which creates a potential for conflicting interests—especially where there is a question of potential culpability or peer review considerations.

In theory, if the organization is ready and committed to patient participation, physicians and employees should feel at ease with the concept. But that is not always the situation. Fear of the unknown is often based on subjective opinions or previous experiences. This fear can inhibit the readiness of some caregivers to accept patient participation in an SFA.

Figure 7-1. Decision Tree to Assist in Judging Patient/Family Readiness

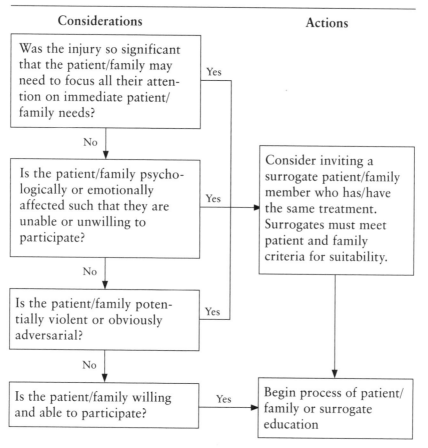

Source: Adapted from T. Zimmerman and G. Amori, "Including Patients in Root Cause Analysis and System Failure Analysis: Legal and Psychological Implications," *Journal of Healthcare Risk Management* 27, no. 2 (2007): 27–34. Copyright ©2007 American Society for Healthcare Risk Management of the American Hospital Association. Used with permission.

Figure 7-2.   Patient Preparation Discussion Elements

Minimum Elements to Discuss with Patients prior to Their Involvement in the System Failure Analysis

Root Cause Analysis Process

- Description of the process
- Goals of the meeting
- Reason the organization uses root cause analysis for process improvement
- What the organization hopes to learn
- What the organization will do with the information
- How the organization will ensure that improvements occur
- Description of the types of people who will participate

Patient's Role in the Process

- Unique contributions of the patient to the process
  - Perspective that naturally may be different from the those of the caregivers
  - Value of the patient's closeness to the event
  - The patient's desire to ensure that whatever happened will not reccur if there is a way to prevent it
- Nature of the patient's participation
  - Level of participation—whether present only for an opening statement or during the entire process
  - Who will be present
  - Expectations for the patient's contribution
  - Expectations for the activity and behavior of other participants during the patient's presence
  - What will be done with the patient's information
  - What the patient can expect after the meeting
  - What the patient should do if he or she feels the meeting has not gone as planned, he or she is uncomfortable, or he or she changes his or her mind about participation

Figure 7-2. (Continued)

Expectations of Patients during and after the Process

- Open and honest communication between patient and caregivers
  - —Behave in respectful manner
  - —Avoid sarcasm, intimidating actions or words, and disruptive or threatening behaviors
- Honor the integrity of the process
  - —Promise not to tape or secretly photograph the meeting
  - —Promise not to use the meeting to gather information that will be used "against" the organization or caregivers
- Recognize that the caregivers are sad and upset
  - —Don't blame or verbally assault caregivers during the meeting
  - —Don't argue about patient care during the meeting

Source: Adapted from T. Zimmerman and G. Amori, "Including Patients in Root Cause Analysis and System Failure Analysis: Legal and Psychological Implications," *Journal of Healthcare Risk Management* 27, no. 2 (2007): 27–34. Copyright © 2007 American Society for Healthcare Risk Management of the American Hospital Association. Used with permission.

Furthermore, the caregiver's sadness and psychological trauma associated with being involved in an adverse event can trigger feelings of vulnerability and guilt. Although system failure is quite likely the root cause of the event, some caregiver participants may feel personally responsible for the incident. This emotion can cripple their ability to effectively participate in the SFA.

Involving patients in an SFA has complex psychological, legal, and emotional implications. Therefore, it is essential that the subject be introduced to caregivers in a positive, educational, and supportive manner. Assurances must be made by the organization that information from the SFA will not be used surreptitiously to fuel peer review, to take unwarranted punitive actions, or to transfer liability away from the organization onto the practitioner. Be sure that caregivers understand that patients will have been screened for readiness prior to participation and adequately prepared to ensure open and nonthreatening discourse during the meeting.

Screen for Readiness

It is essential that caregiver participants, just like patients, be evaluated for psychological readiness. The success of the SFA will be jeopardized if one or more caregivers strongly believe that the patient's perspective is not valuable or the patient should not be involved due to legal ramifications. Further, self-flagellating beliefs about the cause of the event can trigger practitioner guilt that leads to an inappropriate admission of fault before the system failures are uncovered. Conversely, if practitioners believe the event was evitable, regardless of the care provided, patients may view this as an insensitive, uncaring attitude. Caregivers with these beliefs should not be automatically excluded from participating in an SFA that involves the patient; however, the facilitator must anticipate and skillfully manage the potentially disruptive impact of these beliefs on meeting discussions. After the meeting, it is also important that the meeting leader or facilitator carefully debrief caregiver participants who appeared skeptical or resistant to ensure they are emotionally steady with the proceedings.

A second consideration for caregivers is their level of psychological fragility. If a caregiver is unable to come to grips with feelings of guilt or sadness following a catastrophic event, they are probably not good candidates for participation in SFA discussions. In these situations, consider inviting another health care participant with similar experience, education, and background to participate.

Prepare the Caregivers

Health care participants must be emotionally and psychologically capable of providing a safe environment for patient/family participation in the SFA. During meetings, caregivers should behave in an open and respectful manner. Sarcasm, intimidating actions or words, or disruptive and threatening behaviors must be avoided. Achieving this goal will require some pre-meeting preparation. Caregivers must understand that their role is not to challenge the patient but to be supportive and seek additional information that will benefit the process. Open discussion of unanticipated events with the injured party places caregivers in a potentially vulnerable and tenuous situation; thus it is important to address their fears and questions gently and with respect. Caregiver preparation must include sharing information about all of the elements listed in figure 7-3.

When the key stakeholder groups have been carefully screened and adequately prepared for patient participation in an SFA, the process can be a truly valuable and enlightening experience for everyone involved. The narrative in the appendix to this chapter, based on an actual SFA that included patient involvement, illustrates how powerful the experience can be.

Alternatives for Patient Participation

It can be a scary and intimidating experience for patients to be involved in an SFA after having been harmed by an adverse event. The experience can also be scary and intimidating for caregivers. To minimize the psychological impact for everyone, it is often helpful to first experiment with patient participation following a near-miss situation (e.g., wrong medication dispensed but not administered to the patient; wrong body part prepped for surgery, but error was caught and corrected by surgical team during time-out). This limits some of the fears and liability concerns that caregivers may have following a harmful event while at the same time providing the organization with an opportunity to fine-tune the patient participation process. The learning derived from patient involvement in analysis of a near miss can be used by the organization to ready patient and caregiver participants for investigations of more harmful events.

Organizations clearly unable or unwilling to include patients in the entire SFA process should consider alternative strategies for obtaining patient input. Some alternatives are described in the next section. These approaches assume that the recommendations made throughout this chapter are considered here as well.

Figure 7-3.   Caregiver Preparation Discussion Elements

Minimum Elements to Discuss with Caregivers prior to Their Involvement in the System Failure Analysis

Information about the Patient's Role in the Process

- Value of the patient's perspective
- Psychology of the patient's commitment to improving the process
- Nature and level of patient participation in the process
- Legal considerations and how they have been addressed by the organization
- How the patient has been prepared for participation

Caregivers' Role in the Process

- How to behave to preserve the faltering trust and concerns of the patient
- Nonverbal and verbal strategies to ensure caregivers do not inadvertently create tension for the patient
- How the meeting will be structured to ensure the patient feels welcome and comfortable

Expectations of Caregivers during and after the Process

- Open and honest communication between patient and caregivers
    —Behave in respectful manner
    —Avoid sarcasm, intimidating actions or words, and disruptive or threatening behaviors
- Honor the integrity of the process
    —Promise not to tape or secretly photograph the meeting
    —Promise not to use the meeting to gather information that will be used "against" the patient or other caregivers
- Recognize that the patient is sad and upset
    —Don't blame or verbally assault the patient during the meeting
    —Don't argue about patient care during the meeting

Source: Adapted from T. Zimmerman and G. Amori, "Including Patients in Root Cause Analysis and System Failure Analysis: Legal and Psychological Implications," *Journal of Healthcare Risk Management* 27, no. 2 (2007): 27–34. Copyright ©2007 American Society for Healthcare Risk Management of the American Hospital Association. Used with permission.

Limited SFA Participation

If, for whatever reason, the patient is unable to participate in the full SFA, it can be helpful to invite the patient to deliver an "opening statement" at the start of the process. The patient meets with the SFA team at the first meeting for the sole purpose of providing his or her personal perspective surrounding the event. If this approach is used, it is best if the meeting is brief with all participants present. Introduction of the event and the patient should be respectfully and professionally handled. The patient does need to understand beforehand that some of the caregivers in the meeting may have been personally involved in the incident, but these individuals should not be singled out during introductions. All participants, including the patient, will have a certain amount of emotional fragility, so be sure to set the tone at the start by explaining that care, respect, and concern are the expected code of conduct.

The patient may either recount his or her story from memory or read a statement he or she has prepared. The only questions that are permitted from other participants are those intended to clarify the patient's perceptions. Defer open discussion among participants until the next meeting when the patient will not be present. At the close of the patient's statement, it is best if all parties adjourn at the same time. Otherwise, the patient may feel left out or dismissed if escorted from the room prior to the end of the meeting. Experience has shown that having the patient leave the meeting before the rest of the participants creates feelings of separateness and concerns that "they are talking about me now."

If well handled, even limited participation by the patient can be influential in encouraging caregivers to focus on the person and not just the problem. It allows an opportunity for apology and appreciation to be expressed in a group setting. If the dialogue is appropriate and sincerely felt, it can be the starting point of the closure process for everyone involved. Often the patient's opening statement creates a powerful impetus for system improvement spurred by story telling and fueled by human emotion.

Other Input Options

If the patient is unwilling or unable to participate in any part of the SFA process, it is still important to have his or her perspective represented. One way to do this is to interview the patient. The person conducting the interview (perhaps the organization's patient advocate) then presents the patient's story to the SFA team. Other alternatives include reading a statement prepared by the patient or having a video and/or voice recording of the patient telling his or her own story.

Another partnership alternative is to invite the patient to meet with key SFA participants sometime after the analysis has been completed. A patient meeting can provide additional insights into the system improvement plans that are being implemented. Such a meeting can also help the patient see that the organization has taken the injury seriously and is doing something to prevent similar incidents in the future. Just like patient involvement in the SFA itself, this meeting must be carefully and sensitively handled. Also, be sure to seek advice from legal counsel and risk management before scheduling this meeting.

In lieu of asking the patient personally affected by an adverse event to be involved in the SFA, some organizations include a "surrogate" patient—someone who has experienced similar health care services but did not have an adverse event. This allows for the patient perspective to be heard by caregivers. It is recommended that the surrogate patient's treatment be completed before including him or her in the SFA.[16] This will reduce the likelihood that the analysis experience is anxiety producing for the patient—making him or her fearful that a serious event might occur some time during continuing treatment at the facility.

When patient participation in an SFA is not possible due to organizational, patient, or caregiver challenges, other methods of obtaining patient input for system analysis purposes may be used. Patient participants can be invited to attend quality or patient safety committee meetings, where they can provide constructive patient-focused insights. Some organizations have invited patients who experienced a near miss or an adverse event to serve on a patient safety advisory committee, to serve on the board of trustees, or to participate in unit patient safety rounds. These tactics reinforce to caregivers the value and importance of patient-focused care.

Improving Systems Together

The mere suggestion that patients and family members can be involved in an SFA will likely result in an outcry of reasons why it can't or shouldn't be done. All of these reasons have some basis in reality and must not be taken lightly. Health care organizations and caregivers are at a pivotal point in the movement toward patient-centered care and public transparency. We can choose to move forward and manage the fears and risks as much as possible, or we can view the challenges as nonnegotiable barriers and retreat to the more comfortable status quo. The first choice is understandably scary for the organization as well as caregivers. The second choice, although an easier one to make, limits our potential for even greater system safety improvements.

Thankfully, some pioneering health care organizations are already inviting patients and family members to participate in SFAs. Strategies that have worked best at these organizations and how to handle the inevitable challenges are described earlier in this chapter.

Keys for success include adequate preparation of key stakeholders and careful screening of all participants. Even when all precautions are taken, unanticipated situations can occur. The SFA facilitator must be prepared to handle these situations. For example, what if discussions take a negative turn? Should the meeting be promptly ended, or can something be said or done to change the tone in the room? What if the patient or any participant shows up at the meeting with legal counsel? What if someone brings a recorder or camera into the meeting room or secretly records or photographs the meeting without the group's knowledge? What will be done after the meeting to address the continuing emotional needs of the patient and the caregivers involved in the process?

While all of these issues need to be cautiously and thoughtfully considered, none of them should dissuade an organization from considering inclusion of a patient in the SFA process. The positive impact of patient involvement is immeasurable. The organization's first few attempts may not run as smoothly as hoped for, but don't let that dissuade people from continuing the practice. It is the right thing to do for the organization and well worth it for the caregivers and our patients.

References

1. All names have been changed to protect the confidentiality of involved parties. This story is paraphrased from a patient's experiences that were shared with the authors in the course of their practice. Permission was granted by the patient to include this story in the book.
2. Paul Starr, *The Social Transformation of American Medicine* (Jackson, TN: Basic Books, 1949), 4.
3. Ibid.
4. Jody Halpern, *From Detached Concern to Empathy* (New York: Oxford Press, 2001), 16.
5. Institute for Family-Centered Care (Bethesda, MD) [http://www.familycenteredcare.org]. Accessed August 5, 2007.
6. R. J. Blendon, C. M. DesRoches, M. Brodie, J. M. Benson, A. B. Rosen, E. Schneider, D. E. Altman, K. Zapert, M. J. Herrmann, and A. E. Steffenson, "Views of Practicing Physicians and the Public on Medical Errors," *New England Journal of Medicine* 347, no. 24 (2002): 1933–40.
7. John Banja, "Persisting Problems in Disclosing Medical Error," *Harvard Policy Review* 5, no. 1 (2004): 14–19.
8. H. B. Beckman, K. M. Markakis, A. L. Suchman, and R. M. Frankel, "The Doctor-Patient Relationship and Malpractice. Lessons from Plaintiff Depositions," *Archives of Internal Medicine* 154, no. 12 (1994): 1365–70.
9. N. Legros and J. D. Pinkell, "The New JCAHO Patient Safety Standards and the Disclosure of Unanticipated Outcomes," *Journal of Health Law* 35, no. 2 (2002): 189–210.

10. Rae M. Lamb, D. M. Studdert, R. M. Bohmer, D. M. Berwick, and T. A. Brennan, "Hospital Disclosure Practices: Results of a National Survey," *Health Affairs* 22, no. 2 (2003): 73–83.
11. D. Wojcieszak, J. Banja, and C. Houk, "The Sorry Works! Coalition: Making the Case for Full Disclosure," *Joint Commission Journal on Quality and Patient Safety* 32, no. 6 (2006): 344–50; R. C. Boothman, "Apologies and a Strong Defense at the University of Michigan Health System," *Physician Executive* 2, no. 7 (2006): 7–10.
12. B. Raphael and S. Wooding, "Debriefing: Its Evolution and Current Status," *Psychiatric Clinics of North America* 27, no. 3 (2004): 407–23.
13. Patrice L. Spath, "Taming the Measurement Monster," *Frontiers of Health Services Management* 23, no. 4 (2007): 3–14.
14. Raphael and Wooding, "Debriefing: Its Evolution and Current Status."
15. David M. Munch, "As I See It: Patients and Families Can Offer Key Insights in Root Cause Analysis," *Focus on Patient Safety* 7, no. 4 (2004): 6–7.
16. C. M. van Tilburg, I. P. Leistikow, C. M. Rademaker, M. B. Bierings, and A. T. van Dijk, "Health Care Failure Mode and Effect Analysis: A Useful Proactive Risk Analysis in a Pediatric Oncology Ward," *Quality and Safety in Health Care* 15, no. 1 (2006): 58–64.

System Failure Analysis:
An Illustration

"The silence in the room was palpable. The heartfelt sorrow, and the air of forgiveness and understanding, is undeniable."[1]

Mary Ann is recounting a story that affects those involved to this very day. It is a story that the family has continued to live with, a story the staff have relived with patients exhibiting similar symptoms, and a story the risk manager feels proud to have been given the opportunity in which to participate.

Caring for George

George, a man in his early sixties, is a retired railroad worker. He loves the outdoors, is very handy, and is an avid sportsman. His favorite sport is fishing. His sole occupation in life is caring for his wife of many years, who is at home with progressive Alzheimer's disease.

George has lived hard, and his heart took note. He is admitted to the hospital for a coronary artery bypass graft (CABG). He is at a prestigious hospital where a high volume of CABG surgeries are performed. The providers are known for their expertise at harvesting radial arteries for CABG procedures. Although not the typical process used by providers (most harvest veins, not arteries), caregivers at this hospital have many years of experience, and outcome data substantiate their successes. They have never had a bad outcome, and George is confident, trusting, and ready.

The day after surgery, George complains of pain in his left arm. On assessment, his arm is found to be marginally discolored, but not alarmingly so. Throughout the day, George continues to complain of pain. Doppler evaluation of his left arm is inconclusive.

The surgeon, Dr. Sam, is notified. He visits George three times that day, noting his assessment each time in George's medical record. The arm is definitely discolored. At the end of the day, Dr. Sam takes George back to the operating room for a much needed embolectomy.

Back at the intensive care unit that night, the blood flow in George's arm is better. The embolectomy has been effective. Nonetheless, the arm becomes very discolored. Throughout the night, George complains of pain, but it seems more tolerable than before surgery, so caregivers attribute it to normal postoperative pain. By morning, George's arm pain is significant, the pulses are gone, and the discoloration is worse.

Dr. Sam visits George, charts his findings in the medical record, and then leaves. By the end of the second day, George's arm is mottled and cold. The prognosis is clear. George's heart is fine; however, his arm will have to go. Dr. Sam advises George's son, Tim, of the need for amputation.

Failing George and His Family

The effect on Tim is devastating. It's not just that the outcome isn't what he expected. It's that Tim is helpless to do anything. His dad took care of everyone in the family, and now it's Tim's turn to care for his dad. In George's greatest hour of need, Tim feels helpless, hopeless, and frightened. He can't make it right for his dad just like his dad had made it right for him so many times.

In the midst of the chaos, George asks Tim to transcribe a letter addressed to his family. George states that he is about to lose his arm from a complication. "It's part of life," he says. "Please accept it. Don't fight it." George says that he is comfortable that everything will work out. His heart is fine. He also asks that the kids not blame the doctor or the hospital. According to George, this is simply the journey the Lord has set out for him.

The letter goes out by e-mail to George's six children. The family takes a proactive approach to being involved in George's care. They accept the need for an amputation and raise questions about whether an amputation above or below the elbow is better for future functionality of his arm. They ask what is the best way to preserve the most use of his arm. While George is asking his children to forgive those who failed him, the hospital fails him again. Although George and his children are asking for information about various types of amputation, their questions never get answered.

While performing the arm amputation, Dr. Sam becomes increasingly alarmed. He clearly sees what went wrong during the embolectomy. Despite successful removal of the embolus, there was an unseen problem. The stump of the artery is slowly leaking and bleeding into the arm. A distraught Dr. Sam visits the chief of staff. "We found the embolus," he says. "I thought we'd fixed the problem. I had no idea the stump was bleeding."

The disclosure to George and Tim is tough and painful. "We didn't expect this outcome and we never saw it coming."

Participating in Root Cause Analysis

Tim calls the risk manager a few days later asking to talk about the incident. He also wants to share George's letter to the family with her. It is at this point that she brings up the possibility of participation in the root cause analysis (RCA).

George, Tim, and two of Tim's siblings want to participate. After extensive preparation of George and his children and the entire root cause analysis team, this group of fifteen people sit quietly while the risk manager sets the stage for the meeting that is about to start. She has prepped the family and the staff. Some of the premeeting sessions with the staff had not gone well, and the risk manager is nervous. The staff are also nervous. They feel threatened and vulnerable. The hospital has not permitted families to participate in an RCA previously.

Were they being set up for abuse or attack by the family or the organization? They didn't know what to expect.

After setting the stage, the risk manager asks Tim to take the lead in sharing the family's experience. He tells the story from his perspective with input from George and the other siblings. Each person has a unique aspect of the story to share based on when they were present or, in George's case, how alert he was at the time. The family had taken notes during George's hospitalization and refers to these throughout the meeting to make sure they represent the sequence of events accurately. Their attention to detail is admirable. Not surprisingly, emotions run high as their story comes to the end.

After the family shares their story, the staff are asked by the risk manager to reflect on what they experienced. Clearly new information is being shared that carries clues as to what had happened. If these clues had been noticed by the caregivers at the time, the previously presumed unavoidable event might have been prevented. Reactions of the staff are varied. Some accept and embrace the display of emotions and even struggle with their own, while others cross their arms and sit silently.

The quality director then speaks up. "George, I have a message for you from the nurse who cared for you. She was too devastated to be here. She asked me to deliver an apology on her behalf for not being as strong an advocate as she could have been." You could have heard a pin drop in the room. The risk manager feels proud, especially given the dubious attitude of staff during premeeting conversations.

Then it is Dr. Sam's turn. In a very humbling and quiet voice, he leads the caregivers and the family through a journey of George's care. He describes previous conversations with the family. Then silence—the journey changes. Dr. Sam expresses appreciation for the family, their understanding, their willingness to participate, their willingness to share. And then he stops. "And I know you heard me say this already, but I want to tell you again how sorry I am. I was clueless."

The insurance carrier sitting in the room is stunned. The silence in the room is palpable. The heartfelt sorrow, and the air of forgiveness and understanding, is undeniable.

The risk manager brings the meeting to an end, thanking everyone for their openness and honesty. She expresses gratitude to the family for their courage in sharing their story and promises to let them know the outcome of the analysis. The entire group leaves the room together.

Helping George and His Family

In later conversations with the risk manager, the family requests an arm prosthesis for George and help in caring for his wife. In addition, they ask for assistance in modifying the home environment so George can remain as independent as possible. The items requested aren't unreasonable—things like a one-handed can opener.

The most significant request comes at the end of their list. The family wants George to be outdoors again, doing what he loves to do—fishing. He really wants a one-armed rowboat and a launch to match.

It is a small price to pay.

Reference

1. This story is based on an actual event experienced by the authors in the course of their practice. All names have been changed for confidentiality purposes.

8

A Call to Action:
The Leader's Role in Patient Safety

Thomas C. Royer, MD

The goal of excellent patient care is either explicitly expressed or clearly implied in the mission, vision, and value statements of most health care institutions today. To attain this goal, leadership must "walk the talk" and create an environment and culture in which strides to achieve excellence are made every day. Our leadership training teaches excellence, our practitioners strive for it, and our patients and their families deserve it. Leaders of the health delivery process have the responsibility and therefore must be accountable to ensure that the highest quality of care is being delivered to each and every person who enters our doors.

Although creating the vision for excellence may at first seem easy, bringing it to fruition requires a great deal of effort. One explanation is that neither the public nor practicing physicians have a sense of urgency about patient safety and medication errors, according to numerous studies. This is a concern of many national consumer-activist organizations. In fact, according to one recent survey, neither physicians nor the public consider medical errors a significant problem in health care today.[1]

Role of Health Care Leaders

So how do health care leaders make excellence a reality? Hospital chief executive officers and medical directors should take an active interest in patient safety initiatives and support efforts to engage physicians, associate staff, patients, and families in the process. Focused and constant attention is the currency of leadership. Many people will follow if leaders make safety walk-arounds, endorse nonpunitive reporting, and work with the medical executive committee to address issues of poor physician performance. In addition, leadership must encourage open, candid conversations about safety, not only with staff at all levels of the organization but with patients and their families as well. This feedback can be obtained during "real time" rounds or retrospectively, with randomly chosen focus groups. Possible questions to ask in these focus groups include the following:

- Are all caregivers identifying themselves to you?
- Is each person you encounter explaining what he or she is trying to do with you?
- Do you feel trust or confidence in your caregivers?
- Are there times when you have not felt safe? When?
- Would you recommend these services to a friend?
- What could we do to make you feel more secure?

The information received and the suggestions made should be broadly communicated and become a part of the planning process so that appropriate corrective action plans can be put into place.

Consistent Communication

Both verbal and written communications articulated often and consistently must be utilized to elevate patient safety to its appropriate level of importance. This can be accomplished through internal communications to staff members and physicians as well as to patients, using patient education materials or information placed in hospital billing statements. To promote accountability, measurable goals for each of these tactics should be developed and included in annual performance appraisal goals. These should, in part, drive any annual merit increase and also be integrated into any incentive or pay-at-risk programs available to leadership teams. In addition, these communication activities should be incorporated into the organization's annual strategic planning goals. Examples of such strategies include the following:

- Patient safety activities are identified and implemented in all departments and facilities.
- Education materials to facilitate employee focus on improving patient safety are developed and incorporated into the orientation program for new employees.
- A patient safety suggestion box for patients and families is placed in a high-traffic area in both inpatient and out-patient facilities.

Strategic Planning

An effective strategic planning effort allows health care leadership and their staff to design and implement a solid medication safety and patient safety plan. It is imperative that a risk assessment first be done to identify areas where process improvement is needed. Patients and families should be included in these assessments, with input obtained through follow-up phone calls or brief written surveys. Information obtained from such follow-ups in my organization has included the following:

- No one checked my armband before I was given medication.
- A puddle of water on my floor was not cleaned quickly.
- I did not have the opportunity to ask questions of the caregiver before a procedure was done.
- No one explained clearly what the medication I was given was supposed to do.

The information obtained from follow-ups is used to identify specific issues that will need to be incorporated into strategic goals and operating initiatives with clearly defined timelines and responsibilities.

Governance Oversight

Ultimately, accountability for not-for-profit health care delivery systems and public for-profits lies in the governance process. The organization's board of directors should have responsibility for quality oversight and either directly or indirectly (for example, as part of a quality committee) evaluate patient safety data on a regular basis. The board should likewise monitor patient involvement by assessing patient satisfaction scores at least quarterly.

Patient safety measurements should be included in the board's quality report. These measures should be identical to those being reviewed on a regular basis by management to determine if management is meeting its patient satisfaction goals. Clearly, the board report, at a minimum, should include the following:

- Medication errors
- Wrong-site surgeries
- Near-miss incidents
- Falls
- Puncture/needle wounds
- Equipment failures

But more important than identifying the "failures" is clearly articulating what action plans are being implemented to prevent errors from recurring in the future.

Operational Tactics

Clearly, excellence in patient safety will only be achieved if plans are implemented to achieve measurable outcomes within a set period. These operational tactics, which must be strongly supported by leadership, include a wide variety of approaches that can be customized to the individual organization. The most helpful include creating champions, sharing data, developing incentives for patient involvement, education, and supporting external evaluation.

Creating Champions

First and foremost, "champions" must be identified. These are credible, well-respected individuals who clearly understand the issues and possess sufficient energy and focus to lead the corrective action planning and implementation process. Patient safety improvement responsibilities should be incorporated into the job description of these champion staff members. Appropriate educational courses must be offered to expand the patient safety knowledge of the champions. In addition, networks in which they can share and develop best practices should be created.

A patient safety advisory council is most beneficial in helping the operational champions identify issues and find solutions. Membership on this advisory council should be multidisciplinary, consisting primarily of patients and consumers. The council's activities must be supported by an information technology infrastructure and focus on all patient safety concerns, including the common errors that occur when patients are transferred from one area of the continuum of care to another. This group should review and recommend technology that can minimize errors and near misses and also define data sets that can be audited periodically to verify that continuous improvement is occurring. The goal is to achieve consistent and predictable clinical performance for all patients at all times.

Sharing Data

Once the data are known, they should be shared internally and externally with appropriate staff, quality-focused organizations, and monitoring agencies. Voluntary peer reporting is important to determine best practices as well as to understand the gap between where an organization is presently and where it should be. Once this gap is understood, appropriate tactics must be put in place to achieve excellence. Networking among those with better performance is an ideal way to learn about, and then transplant, practices to make improvements in a "rapid cycle" fashion. In addition, all patients must have access to and "ownership" of their own health data, which, it is hoped, will increase their participation in maintaining health.

Developing Incentives for Patient Involvement

It is also appropriate to develop incentives, both monetary and otherwise, to heighten patients' participation in medication safety and standardization of care. These might include rewards for compliance with drug regimens and disease management programs. Rewards should include products that are health related; successful examples include the following:

- Car seats for children
- Free or discounted physical exams
- Discounts on vitamins
- Free or discounted childhood immunizations
- Sessions in exercise clubs
- Free classes on nutrition
- Free classes on smoking cessation

Educating Patients, Families, and Staff

The leadership team should also be supportive of the development of educational programs that highlight ways that patients and their families can collaborate with caregivers to ensure a safe health care environment, safe processes, and safe procedures. Patients should be encouraged to ask questions, compiled beforehand, and providers should listen carefully and answer them. Patients should also be encouraged to bring all medications to the encounter, as well as a copy of their advance directive. Any instructions, including information about medications, should be given in the language a patient can understand, and prescription labeling should be clear and distinct.

While in the hospital, patients should receive constant reminders to make sure all members of their caregiver team are aware of patients' important personal health information, such as allergies or chronic conditions. Also, patients should feel free to question medication and tests as they would in an outpatient setting. All of this information is extremely helpful and can be included in a patient guidebook.

The guidebook would remind patients to actively participate in ensuring their own safety. Patients should be encouraged to ask all caregivers if they are familiar with patients' allergies and the combination of medicines patients are taking. Patients should also be made aware of major safety hazards, such as not having assistance when medicated, falling over equipment that clutters the space around the bed, or being asked to take medicine left at the bedside. A whiteboard in each patient's room, where the patient, family, and caregivers can easily view it, is also an excellent method of recording data to enhance the safety environment for the patient.

The name of the major caregivers by shift, as well as the patient's allergies, should be clearly available to all caregivers coming to the bedside. The patient's chronic conditions and medications can also be included on the board; however, especially in light of Health Insurance Portability and Accountability Act privacy regulations, the patient's consent must first be given. The more this type of information is consistently available, the safer the environment will be.

Supporting External Evaluation

Although doing so is at times challenging, health care leaders should also support external accrediting bodies that survey any aspect of patient safety. The findings of such surveys may contain some controversial issues at times, but this feedback provides one more set of eyes to evaluate performance, identify gaps between reality and goals, and offer advice for improvement. The continuous improvement mentality that the outside review process creates in a facility is a positive halo effect in moving the organization to a higher level of patient safety and improved quality.

Making Excellence Commonplace

Health care leaders carry an awesome responsibility, because patients entering our doors are placing their life—their most precious gift—in our hands. Consequently, we must strive to care for each person in an excellent manner, ensuring that the treatment environment is as safe as possible. By collaborating with patients, families, and staff and listening to suggestions, the leadership team can make continual improvements, which is why it is imperative to tap into the insightful perspectives and creative solutions of our stakeholders. More often than not, the information gleaned proves to be a valuable resource in improving safety and reducing medication errors, thereby improving the overall quality and outcome of care. In the end, we should be so confident in our ability to provide a truly safe environment—one in which excellence is commonplace—that we could offer a service guarantee to each person who walks through our doors. Otherwise, we should "pay the penalty" and rapidly institute a corrective action plan so we will achieve success in the future.

A "service guarantee" environment demands a strong team effort from staff, as well as an intense focus on getting patients and their families involved as additional safeguards in the system. Patients must be involved in education processes focusing on patient safety issues in their encounters, readily accepted as active participants in maintaining their safety during their encounters, and questioned after their encounters to understand what made them feel safe and then listen to their suggestions as to what improvements could be made. Specific examples of how to accomplish these goals are highlighted in this chapter.

On an ongoing basis, the progress in improving the health care environment so that it is providing cost-efficient and effective care delivered with the highest degree of safety possible can be monitored by periodically receiving and reviewing the following information at both the management and governance levels:

- Patient satisfaction scores
- Associate and employee satisfaction scores

- Physician satisfaction scores
- Medication error rate
- Near-miss incidents
- Measurements of agreed-on quality metrics
- Patient falls
- Complaints
- Legal/risk claims
- Puncture wounds from needles
- Equipment failures
- Nosocomial infections

Every health care organization must have clearly articulated, measurable goals for patient safety. Goal attainment should be regularly monitored so that continuous improvement can be made toward creating a safe and pleasant environment for each patient who enters our doors.

Reference

1. R. J. Blendon, C. M. DesRoches, M. Brodie, J. M. Benson, A. B. Rosen, E. Schneider, D. E. Altman, K. Zapert, M. J. Herrmann, and A. E. Steffenson, "Views of Practicing Physicians and the Public on Medical Errors," *New England Journal of Medicine* 347, no. 24 (2002): 1965–67.

9

Royal Oak Beaumont Hospital: Putting the Patient in Patient Safety

Kay Beauregard and Steven Winokur, MD

Royal Oak Beaumont Hospital in Royal Oak, Michigan, is a large (1,061 beds) community teaching hospital and a member of the Association of American Medical Colleges Council of Teaching Hospitals. In 2006, for the eleventh year in a row, Beaumont received the National Research Corporation Consumer Choice Award for the "most preferred hospital" in southeastern Michigan. Achieving this distinction has been in part due to the organization's continuing commitment to embracing patients (and family/support groups) as active and informed healthcare partners.

Laying the Groundwork

The Beaumont board of directors has always made patient safety a top priority. In 2000, the board reaffirmed this commitment by identifying patient safety as the guiding principle in achieving quality. The board demonstrates support for patient safety through executive appointments, sufficient personnel, requests for patient safety outcome information, and resource allocation. In January 2001, Beaumont established its Patient Safety Council. The council, composed of corporate leaders, medical staff, and quality leaders and the Department of Legal Affairs, oversees all patient safety activities. The board of directors appointed a physician leader as chief patient safety officer in 2001.

The organization's leadership demonstrates that patient safety is a top priority by communicating with employees and medical staff at all levels, encouraging active involvement of staff and physicians on patient safety committees, and educating employees about safety-related issues. The revised employee orientation program includes patient safety, and department managers' meetings routinely include items that relate to patient safety.

The sheer size of the hospital and scope of the patient safety program created a challenge in reaching all medical staff and employees. Implementing change throughout all levels of the organization required a unique blend of committed leadership, networking, and empowerment of patient safety advocates throughout the organization. Complex organizational theory has been extremely helpful in designing the approach to changing our culture.

A Supportive Culture

Beaumont has a long-standing tradition of pursuit of clinical excellence, quality improvement, and outcomes measurement. Commitment to education includes training programs in the following areas:

- Graduate medical education
- Medical student education with formal medical school affiliations
- Nursing education
- Pharmacy education
- Radiology education

Beaumont is integrating the culture of safety through its leadership, education and training programs, allocation of resources, and personnel sufficient to ensure a state-of-the-art capability for process improvement.

Reporting is promoted by offering multiple paths by which participants can report an error or near miss, including written patient safety and quality improvement (PSQI) reports or an anonymous hotline. A nonpunitive environment for error reporting is demonstrated by the responses to reported errors. Process owners (recipients of variance reports) send thank you letters to staff or physicians who have reported errors. Recognition programs, such as wow cards, are given to staff members who participate in patient safety rounds. Wow cards are the size of a business card and are redeemable in the various hospital retail settings.

The human resources department provides education and support to managers for ensuring that staff involved in errors have appropriate assistance and are not penalized. Counseling and support services are available to all employees and medical staff who might need to overcome feelings of grief, frustration, anger, embarrassment, guilt, or loss of confidence that may occur as a result of clinical error. Incorporating "patient safety storytelling" has been effective in promoting candid discussion. Staff members who see genuine process change as a result of their reports will continue to report.

Process improvement teams composed of process owners develop and implement risk-reduction action plans to prevent recurrences of similar events. Action plans are continually evaluated for effectiveness based on data. Patients are asked to provide feedback regarding patient safety. Specific instructions are given to patients on partnering with caregivers to provide safe care. Patients and families have a dedicated phone line on which to report safety concerns, and they learn about the phone line from printed material, such as the "You and Your Caregivers: Partners in Safety" brochure that is described later in this chapter. The phone line is the same one publicized in the bedside patient guide and other informational brochures for dealing with patient concerns. The phone line connects patients to the Service Excellence department, whose personnel handle calls promptly and involve the unit manager and other appropriate personnel. Although the phone line is available for use during the hospital stay, many patients and families prefer to call after discharge.

Policies That Form the Foundation

Various policies were developed or revised to support the patient safety infrastructure and reflect patient safety as our guiding principle in achieving quality. Policies support such concepts as recognition of human errors as inevitable, even among the most conscientious professionals practicing the highest standard of care, and recognition that learning from errors is critical if we are to design safer systems. These policies cover topics such as variance reporting, sentinel event response, and corrective actions.

The chain-of-command policy describes the expectation that staff will report real or potential patient safety issues and the infrastructure to support staff when they do. The informed consent policy describes the expectation that patients will be involved in decision making. A policy called Employees Involved in Clinical Errors was developed to encourage a patient-safe culture. The policy outlines the support process, which is intended to assist employees in resolving such issues as grief, frustration, and embarrassment when they are involved in a clinical error. These policies provide a consistent framework by which all departments can function. They demonstrate a commitment to staff members that the organization will support them as individual practitioners and will focus on providing systems that promote safe care for the patient.

The Impact of Change

The culture change at Beaumont has been observable in a number of different ways, such as the following:

- An increase in error reporting has been documented, including an increase in the reporting of close-call events.
- Discussions of patient safety issues occur at staff meetings on a regular basis.
- Nurses routinely read back orders to physicians.
- Transporters "stop the line" and don't take patients off the unit without an identification band physically attached to all patients.

Processes have changed as a direct result of analysis and prioritization of information learned from PSQI reports, safety rounds, direct communication with frontline staff, and other proactive opportunities. Examples of safety improvement projects include, but are not limited to, the following:

- Make It Complete—guidelines for ordering medication
- What's In a Name—using Tallman lettering for medication safety
- Medication checks and balances—using new guardrails on infusion pumps, for example
- Information transfer during patient handoffs
- Six Sigma's dramatic impact in Central Processing
- Voice-activated wireless communication badges improve telemetry alert response

Current Strengths in Patient Involvement

Beaumont has created a firm foundation of patient safety that has allowed the increased involvement of patients. Several initiatives, described in the following sections, are under way to strengthen and expand this involvement.

Patient and Family Advisory Council

The Patient and Family Advisory Council was established in 2006. The council is composed of Beaumont leadership and staff, as well as members of the community. Approximately fifty members of the community applied to be on the council. Following an interview process, twelve were selected for a two-year team.

The council's mission is to speak as a unified voice for the patients and their visitors at Beaumont. The council helps staff members, physicians, and volunteers understand what it is like to be a patient or visitor. The council also identifies ways to make Beaumont's care and environment more centered on the needs of patients and their visitors and provides an opportunity for patients and families to provide input into policy and program development. Specific patient safety agenda items have included care and communication in the emergency center, design of the "perfect" patient admission, and the patient's and family's role in infection control and hand hygiene.

A council member commentary following a meeting on infection control stated:

They [Beaumont] are doing more than just tracking. They're into preventing infections by means large and small, complex and simple. They monitor procedures in operations rooms. They know what's in the air and what's in the water. They've even got rooms that are designed to prevent contaminated air from entering a hallway when a door is opened. But the simplest thing they are doing is what our mothers taught us: wash our hands. All patient rooms have dispensers that hold a disinfectant solution. Anyone coming in and going out must wash his or her hands. In the fall of 2007, kiosks were installed near the entrance with the same dispensers. Visitors will be encouraged to wash their hands when entering and leaving the hospital.

Patient Education Specialists

The hospital has an educational design department and dedicated education specialists who are accomplished in designing patient education materials that are translated into multiple languages and are adaptable to many situations. The educational design department has developed diverse patient education materials for specific disease categories, equipment use, and therapies; the pain scale, for example, is translated into twenty-one languages.

The department designs communication tools that can be used by family or health care workers to communicate with non–English-speaking or aphasic patients; patient tools are pictures and other methods to enhance communication. Enhanced communication with patients and families results in a greater chance of a safer outcome. During the patient identification process, for example, patients are asked to state their name; to ensure that staff can adequately communicate with all patients, this request has been translated into Arabic (figure 9-1).

Figure 9-1.   Beaumont Hospitals Patient Identification Request, Translated into Arabic

ما إسمك ؟

ما اسمك ؟

What is your name?

Source: Beaumont Hospitals, Royal Oak, Michigan, ©2007. Reprinted with permission.

Recognition of Patient Involvement

The hospital embraces and fosters cultural diversity. Interpreter services are available, as are a large number of clinical pathways, clinical practice guidelines, and patient pathways. Patient versions of pathways help to foster patient safety; these pathways describe for patients the tests, treatments, and therapies that can be expected during their course of stay. Patients are encouraged to question variations from the pathway. For example, if a therapy that is listed on the patient pathway for a specific postoperative day does not occur, the patient can bring this omission to the nurse's attention. If a patient is asked to undergo a diagnostic test that is not listed on the pathway, the patient can question the deviation. Patients' actions may prevent a missed therapy or an inadvertent mistake in the ordering process that could cause a patient to undergo an incorrect diagnostic test.

Inviting Patients to Participate

Efforts to include patients as partners on the health care team include development of a brochure titled "You and Your Caregivers: Partners in Safety." Educational specialists, public relations specialists, physicians, nurses, and other leaders came together to develop a brochure that communicates to patients how they can participate in their own care. It conveys that patients have a role in making health care safe and that patient safety is a top priority for us. The brochure gives the patient specific directions on how to participate in his or her care, such as through the patient identification process, medication process, surgical process, infection control, and other safety tips. Contents of the brochure are found in figure 9-2.

The brochure is included in the packet of information that patients receive on admission and is also mailed to patients prior to outpatient procedures. Physicians and staff members are encouraged to use the information in the brochure to open a discussion with patients about the value of the patients' involvement in care, and it assists the staff in articulating the concept of partnering with patients.

Through the brochure development process, it was discovered that the health care team had different opinions about how the patient could be involved in his or her care. Thus, it was important that implementation of the "You and Your Caregivers" brochure involved patients as well as physicians and staff. Everyone needed to expand his or her understanding of the patient's role in safety. The medical director sent an introductory letter to every physician with a copy of the brochure indicating that patients would be receiving the brochure, and hospital administration sent a similar letter to all department managers indicating that patients would be receiving the brochure—all of which demonstrated leadership support for involvement of the patient. It is expected that caregivers will view a patient's questioning care as providing an opportunity to prevent an error.

As the process evolves, we are learning of more opportunities for patients to participate in their care. For example, on patient safety rounds in the patient registration area, leaders learned that registration clerks have the patient review his or her wristband before it is attached to confirm accuracy. Feedback from our volunteer staff indicates that we need to have the brochure translated into different languages. Furthermore, patients have stated they think the information is good and are pleased to see the hospital is being proactive in its approach to safety.

Figure 9-2. Contents of the "You and Your Caregivers: Partners in Safety" Brochure at Beaumont Hospitals

Everyone has a role in making health care safe: physicians, nurses, pharmacists, technicians . . . and even you! Patient safety is a top priority for Beaumont Hospitals. As the patient, you also play a vital role in safe care by taking an active and informed part.

People come to Beaumont for the excellence of the care—and for the staff who provide that care. In health care, many complex medical procedures are performed daily. Please help your caregiver provide the kind of care you expect from Beaumont.

Please tell us if you have questions or concerns about your care.

- If possible, bring a family member or friend with you. That individual can help you feel more comfortable and help you remember questions you may have or instructions you receive.

- Feel free to ask questions to clarify what a medication is for, what test is going to be performed, or why something is being done.

- You're welcome to call our customer hotline.

Pay attention to the care you are receiving.

- You'll be asked your name and will have your wristband ID checked often during your stay. This will help us identify who you are as we provide care.

- Make sure your nurse or doctor checks your wristband or asks your name before administering any medication or treatment.

- If you're having surgery, you can expect your doctor to mark the area that is to be operated on. Please feel free to ask about it.

- Expect health care workers to introduce themselves when they enter your room. Look for their name badges.

- Illness can spread when individuals do not wash their hands or wear gloves. It's OK to ask those who touch you whether they have washed their hands.

- Tell your nurse or doctor if something doesn't seem quite right.

Know what medications you are taking and why.

- Carry a list of all medications that you take and the amount you take. Include vitamins, herbal supplements, and over-the-counter drugs. This information is important to your caregivers.

- Tell your doctors and nurses about any allergies, side effects, or problems you have had with medications in the past or are currently experiencing.

(Continued on next page)

Figure 9-2.   (Continued)

- We expect questions. Feel free to ask why a medication is being given or if it looks different or unusual to you.

Educate yourself about your diagnosis, the medical tests you are having, and your treatment plan.

- Ask for information about your condition from your doctor or nurse. We often have written booklets, videos, educational TV programs, and information about Web sites and support groups.

- Make sure that information you will need is written down.

- Make sure you know how to use any equipment needed for your care at home after you leave the hospital.

Be a part of all decisions about your treatment.

- Share all information about your medical condition and any special needs with your caregivers.

- Be sure to provide details about your medical history, such as illnesses and operations, as well as symptoms you are having.

- Make sure you understand the information you receive. Ask questions as many times as you need to.

Source: Beaumont Hospitals, Royal Oak, Michigan, ©2007. Reprinted with permission.

Patient Interviews on Safety Rounds

Administrative and management rounds are conducted weekly by administrators, patient safety officers, infection control practitioners, and environmental safety experts in all inpatient and ambulatory settings. More than 100 clinical departments are visited annually. As part of the rounds, the leaders discuss safety with at least one patient to gain feedback from the patient's perspective. The "You and Your Caregivers" brochure is used to guide the conversation, such as by asking the following (or similar) questions:

- Have you noticed the staff asking you to state your name, or have they checked your identification band?

- Have you or your family had a chance to review the information in this brochure?

- If you had surgery, were you asked to mark your surgical site? If so, what do you think about that process?
- Would you feel comfortable asking a doctor if he or she had washed his or her hands before examining you?

The patient safety leaders also use the rounds to model or demonstrate methods for discussing safety issues with patients to assist managers in developing these skills.

Customized Patient Education Materials

The educational design department has developed a process to incorporate patient safety tips when developing materials. If the subject matter expert (author) for the educational materials has not included patient safety information, the patient education specialist will bring this to the author's attention. The authors are referred to the "You and Your Caregivers" brochure as a reference. Other resources, such as those developed by the National Patient Safety Foundation, are also used. Patient educational materials have an approval process that includes departmental, medical, and administrative involvement. For example, in the "Diabetes—What You Need to Know" educational booklet, the safety tips include these:

- Check the label on your insulin bottle to be sure you have the correct type.
- Make sure your insulin syringe and insulin bottle are marked with the same concentration.
- Always read your labels.

Active Patient Involvement

Although the goal is to have active patient involvement in health care processes, caregivers can't expect patients to intuitively know how they can be involved. It is also not expected that patients will know about health care processes or when to question the process. Thus, caregivers are evaluating specific processes to determine how and when to invite the patient to be involved. Physicians and staff members need to prompt and direct patients on how they can be involved.

The point of involvement should be at a critical quality step—the point at which patient involvement in error prevention would be a valued addition. Patient (or family) involvement at a critical quality step adds another layer of safety. The following examples demonstrate practices where active involvement of patients in a specific process is encouraged:

- Patients are involved in the site-marking process for surgery.
- Patients are involved in the patient identification process. A patient actively states his or her first and last name instead of responding to a health care worker who calls out the name. In some instances, patients have been known to respond to an incorrect name. Recently, a patient was asked why he answered to the wrong name, and the patient's comment was, "It was the right time for my test, so I thought it was me."
- Patients participate in the process of protecting children from abductions. Patients are told, "We want to prevent an abduction, and this is how you can help." This statement makes it more real to parents and has been incorporated into our written patient/family educational materials.
- Patients are asked to read and verbally confirm their name and, when available, birth date on materials that are given to them. For example, they may be asked to verify their name on medical records, prescription medications, and radiology studies (x-rays).

Gaining Employee Input

To gain further insight into opportunities for involving patients in their care, employees are being asked to help. A patient safety leader assembled a cross-departmental group and facilitated a roundtable discussion. Recognizing that our employees have also been consumers of health care, we asked them, "How do you check that things are going right when you or a loved one is seeking medical care?" The answers varied:

- A phlebotomist stated, "I ask to see the blood label to verify my name when blood is being drawn, or I may ask to observe that the correct label is being put on the correct tube."
- A pharmacist responded, "I assess the medications my loved one is receiving."
- Another respondent said, "I read the chart, ask questions, mark procedure sites, and educate myself about my condition."

These perspectives are valuable as the organization seeks new opportunities to involve patients in their care. Although this was a one-time exercise, it can be repeated in any patient safety meeting. The exercise demonstrates to staff members that they should personally practice techniques to safeguard against errors and that there is value in teaching patients to do the same.

Continuing Involvement after an Adverse Event

Because trust is paramount and a foundation of patient safety, Beaumont has an active process of disclosure of any event that results in an unanticipated outcome. Beaumont recognizes that after the disclosure the patient and/or family continue to need assistance. Support may be needed to work through an anger or grief process or to understand what the hospital is doing to prevent future occurrences. Pastoral care and social work departments may become actively involved in these situations.

Measuring Success

Evaluating the achievement of patient safety goals is accomplished through direct feedback from frontline care providers, support staff, and patients. Patient safety leaders use patient safety rounds to gather feedback from staff about the effectiveness of the program. Departmental patient safety assessment tools are provided for managers to use in assessing implementation of patient safety interventions.

Beaumont also conducts organization-wide employee and physician surveys to assess patient safety culture, teamwork, error reporting (nonpunitive environment), education, and leadership responsiveness to patient safety issues. The types of information that are gleaned from these surveys are illustrated in figure 9-3. Areas for improvement are identified and assigned to key leaders in the organization. Progress toward resolution is tracked through the hospital's performance improvement structure. Patient safety measures are reported monthly to the board.

Department Data on Patient Safety

A patient safety department assessment tool is used during patient safety rounds (figure 9-4). Managers complete this self-assessment of patient safety efforts within their department. Data are aggregated on each question. Questions specific to patient/family communication include the following:

- Patients are included in safety planning by encouraging them to participate in their care.
- Written materials are provided to patients and families that describe their role as partners in patient safety.
- The department embraces its responsibility and acknowledges its ethical obligation to communicate with patients when unanticipated outcomes have occurred. This includes an explanation of the outcome and its effects, provided in a timely, truthful, and compassionate manner.

Other questions focus on department leadership, creating a learning environment, teamwork and collaboration, and performance measurement.

Figure 9-3. Results of Employee Patient Safety Surveys at Beaumont Hospitals

Question: **When management discovers an employee made a mistake, the employee generally is not punished.***

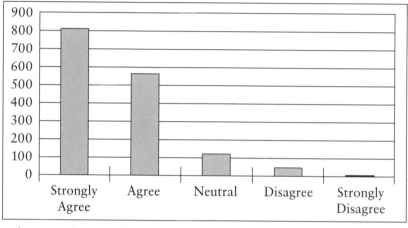

*The vertical axis indicates number of responses. All data are fictitious.

Question: **When I or someone in my work area makes a mistake, we should all know about it so others don't make the same mistake.***

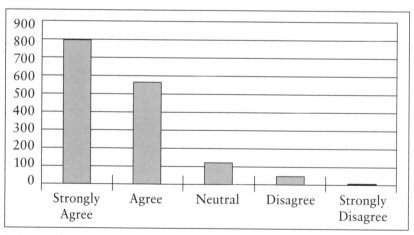

*The vertical axis indicates number of responses. All data are fictitious.

Figure 9-4.   Royal Oak Beaumont Hospital Patient Safety Department Assessment

Place an "X" in the box that most closely represents implementation status.
A = fully implemented throughout the department
B = partially implemented in the department
C = discussed but not implemented
D = no activity

Key Aspect of Safety: Leadership	A	B	C	D
Patient safety goals and objectives are communicated across the department.				
Department leadership regularly monitors and communicates progress in implementing the patient safety initiatives/programs.				
Safety principles are considered when designing and maintaining products/programs/processes.				
Department leaders establish visible commitment to patient safety by participating/performing one or more of the following activities:				
• Periodic observation of routine operations				
• Periodic "walk-arounds" to discuss patient safety and patient safety issues with direct care providers				
Patient safety orientation is provided to all new employees/physicians.				
Employee and medical staff roles and responsibilities in advancing patient safety are appropriately included in job descriptions, orientation, and continuing education.				
Key Aspect of Safety: Creating a Learning Environment	A	B	C	D
The department complies with a nonpunitive policy to address patient adverse events involving medical staff and employees.				
Lessons learned, safe practices, insights, and alerts received from internal and external sources are evaluated and appropriately acted on.				
Recognition and reporting of errors and hazardous conditions are encouraged and rewarded by the department.				

Figure 9-4.   (Continued)

There is a department system of feedback of information about errors and close calls that results in changes and improvements to procedures and/or systems.				
Following a patient safety adverse event, support is provided to involved staff.				
Key Aspect of Safety: Teamwork and Collaboration	A	B	C	D
The department uses checklists, protocols, reminders, decision support, and standardizes equipment, forms, times, and locations to avoid reliance on memory.				
Patient care processes use a minimum number of steps and handoffs.				
Accurate and timely information including clinical results and reference material is available to each clinical decision maker at the point of care.				
Process redesigns and system changes are monitored for effectiveness.				
The department seeks active input from end users of technologies, supplies, and products prior to purchase.				
Interdisciplinary team training, including physicians, is routinely conducted for caregivers.				
Key Aspect of Safety: Patient/Family Communication	A	B	C	D
Patients are included in safety planning by encouraging them to participate in their care.				
Written materials are provided to patients/families that describe their role as partners in patient safety.				
The department embraces its responsibility and acknowledges its ethical obligation to communicate with patients when unanticipated outcomes have occurred. This includes an explanation of the outcome and its effects, provided in a timely, truthful, and compassionate manner.				
Key Aspect of Safety: Measurement	A	B	C	D
Performance outcomes and indicators are established to support and monitor implementation of patient safety plans and measure safety performance.				

Source: Beaumont Hospitals, Royal Oak, Michigan. ©2007. Reprinted with permission.

Hospital Data on Patient Safety

The hospital has a robust system for collecting data about, and analyzing key processes through, our variance reporting structure (known as incident reports in other organizations). Specific problematic processes were initially selected by analyzing historical data about variances. Once the key processes of interest were determined (patient falls, medication events, equipment events, and so on), process owners were recruited. A management engineer, an administrator, and a physician provide support for each process owner.

A standardized system was developed for all process owners to use in assessing, tracking, and analyzing variance data. All process owners evaluate events using a predefined set of potential root cause process breakdowns. Root cause process breakdowns include security systems and processes, the physical environment, equipment, and the patient identification process. Data from all process owner reports are aggregated, so the organization can see improvement opportunities in individual processes as well as opportunities that cross process lines. The information is used to establish safety improvement priorities for the organization. A sample aggregate report of process breakdowns is shown in figure 9-5.

As with any continuous process improvement effort, Beaumont focuses actions on the opportunities identified. The overall results of the patient safety survey show that through employee education programs we are attaining our goal of reinforcing systems to minimize errors, learning from our mistakes, and sharing what we have learned with others while keeping the patient at the center of all we do.

Specific measurement of the impact of patient involvement on error reduction will be difficult to extrapolate from existing data. Patient involvement adds one more safety layer to reduce the risk of errors; thus, the actual events should decrease. The process of patient involvement can be measured through direct observations (for example, did the staff member ask the patient to state his or her name?). To evaluate the impact of the

Figure 9-5. Report of Process Breakdowns Contributing to Variances at Beaumont Hospitals*

Process Breakdown	Number of Reported Breakdowns
Communication among staff members	9
Communication with patient/family	5
Physical assessment process	4
Patient identification process	4
Care planning process	3
Orientation and training of staff	3
Physical environment	3
Availability of information	3
Patient observation process	2
Equipment maintenance or management	2
Staffing levels	2
Labeling of medications	2
Adequacy of technological support	2
Security systems and processes	2
Control of medications: storage/access	1
Competency assessment and credentialing	1
Supervision of staff	1
Continuum of care	1
Behavioral assessment process	0

*The horizontal axis indicates the number of reported breakdowns. All data are fictitious.

Source: Beaumont Hospitals, Royal Oak, Michigan. ©2007. Reprinted with permission.

actual involvement, staff members may be encouraged to report (through existing variance report systems) instances where the patient's involvement prevented an error.

Patients as Partners in Safe Care

It is essential for health care organizations to create a culture of patient safety before jumping in with the expectation that staff will embrace patients as partners in care. The fundamentals of building safe systems, process improvement, learning from errors and close calls, and reducing the fear of inappropriate punitive reactions will build a culture of trust. Staff members who are equipped with the appropriate skills and practice in a supportive culture will more readily embrace the value of having the patient as a partner in care. Organizations that are proactive and teach patients how to be partners in the patient safety movement will have a win-win situation.

Resource List

Numerous resources are available to help patients and their families participate more fully in the health care experience. Below are resources specifically focused on engaging consumers in patient safety. Some of the materials are intended to educate consumers on their role in reducing medical errors, and other resources are for health care professionals seeking ways to improve consumer involvement in safety initiatives. Many of the organizations and companies listed have additional health care quality and safety improvement resources. The number of resources that can be used to engage consumers in patient safety continues to grow every day. A current list of resources is maintained on the Internet at http://www.brownspath.com/.

Health Care Safety Fact Sheets and Other Resources for Consumers

Agency for Healthcare Research and Quality
http://www.ahrq.gov

Consumer fact sheets, videos, brochures (some Spanish versions):

- 20 Tips to Help Prevent Medical Errors
- 5 Steps to Safer Health Care
- Your Guide to Choosing Quality Health Care
- Having Surgery? What You Need to Know
- Improving Health Care Quality: A Guide for Patients and Families
- Ways You Can Help Your Family Prevent Medical Errors
- 20 Tips to Help Prevent Medical Errors in Children

- Check Your Medicines
- Questions Are the Answer: Get More Involved in Your Healthcare (video)

American Academy of Orthopaedic Surgeons
http://orthoinfo.aaos.org

Consumer fact sheets:

- Avoiding an Epidemic of Errors
- How Herbal Supplements Interact with Medications
- Partner with Your Physician for the Best Surgical Outcome
- Patients Have Important Role in Safer Health Care

American Society for Healthcare Risk Management
http://www.ashrm.org/ashrm/foundation/emmisafety/
Emmi.html

- Video on steps consumers can take to get involved in their own health care (Flash player required)

Ask About Medicines
http://www.askaboutmedicines.org/

Consumer brochures:

- Ask about Your Diabetes Medicines
- Ask about Your Cancer Medicines

Association of periOperative Nurses
http://patientsafetyfirst.org

Consumer fact sheets:

- Who's Who in the Hospital
- Finding Surgical Information You Can Trust
- Choosing a Doctor to Do Your Surgery
- What You Need to Know about Your Surgery

- What You Need to Know about Anesthesia
- Advice for Patients Concerned about Correct Site Surgery

Food and Drug Administration
http://www.fda.gov

Consumer fact sheets (Spanish versions available):

- Drug Interactions: What You Should Know
- We Want You to Know about X-Rays: Get the Picture on Protection
- How to Give Medicine to Children
- Medicines and Older Adults
- Use Medicine Safely
- Buying Medicines and Medical Products Online

Hospital & Healthsystem Association of Pennsylvania
http://www.haponline.org

Consumer education videos:

- Medication Safety Practices (video)
- Partnering with Your Physician (video)
- Taking an Active Role in Your Healthcare (video)

Institute for Safe Medication Practices
http://www.ismp.org

Consumer education resources:

- Alerts and Tools for Consumers
- General Advice on Safe Medication Use
- Lessons to Be Learned from Past Errors
- Preventing Drug Errors in Children

Johns Hopkins Hospital Patient Safety Brochure and Video
http://www.hopkinsmedicine.org/patients/safety/index.html

Joint Commission
http://www.jointcommission.org

Consumer fact sheets and brochures:

- Help Prevent Errors in Your Care: For Surgical Patients
- Preparing to Be a Living Organ Donor
- Three Things You Can Do to Prevent Infection
- Things You Can Do to Prevent Medication Mistakes
- Planning Your Recovery
- What You Should Know about Research Studies

Legacy Health System Patient Safety Brochure, "It's OK to Ask"
http://www.legacyhealth.org/documents/Misc/ItsOK.pdf

Madison (WI) Patient Safety Collaborative
http://www.madisonpatientsafety.org

Consumer fact sheets and brochures:

- Using Your Medications Safely: A Guide to Prescription Health
- Pocket Card to Record Medications
- What You Can Do to Partner with Healthcare Professionals to Improve Safety
- Pharmacy Safety and Service
- Preventing Infections in the Hospital—What You Can Do
- The Role of the Patient Advocate
- Safety as You Go from Hospital to Home

Massachusetts Coalition for the Prevention of Medical Errors
http://www.macoalition.org

Consumer brochures:

- Your Role in Safe Medication Use
- Action to Help Protect Yourself
- Medication Safety Advice

My Personal Health Information, sponsored by the American
Health Information Management Association
http://www.myphr.com/

- My Personal Health Record: A Guide to Understanding
  and Managing Your Personal Health Information

National Alliance for Caregiving
http://www.caregiving.org

Consumer education resources:

- Hospital Discharge Planning: Helping Family
  Caregivers through the Process
- A Family Caregiver's Guide to Hospital Discharge
  Planning (Spanish version available)

National Center for Injury Prevention and Control
http://www.cdc.gov/ncipc

Consumer fact sheets:

- Falls and Hip Fractures among Older Adults
- Check for Safety: A Home Fall Prevention Checklist for
  Older Adults

National Council on Patient Information and Education
http://www.talkaboutrx.org

Consumer fact sheets and other education resources (some
Spanish versions):

- Your Medicine: Play It Safe
- Get the Most from Your Medicine: Managing Side Effects
- Get the Answers (wallet card)
- Prescription for Safety (mirror sticker)
- Educate before You Medicate
- Alcohol and Medicine: Ask before You Mix
- Buying Prescription Medicines Online

- Taking the Mystery Out of Managing Your Medicines (video)
- Make Notes & Take Notes to Avoid Medication Errors

National Family Caregivers Association
http://www.nfcacares.org

Tip sheets and how-to guides:

- Speak Up
- Choosing a Nursing Home, A Caregiver's Guide
- Improving Doctor Caregiver Communications
- Checklists for Healthcare Encounters
- Medical Record Form to Keep Track of All Medications
- How to Communicate Your Loved One's Symptoms in a Crisis
- Questions to Ask Your Healthcare Provider
- How to Communicate Your Loved One's Needs about Well-Being, Pain and More

National Institute on Aging
http://www.nia.nih.gov/HealthInformation/Publications

Consumer fact sheets and brochures:

- Medicines: Use Them Safely
- Home Safety for People with Alzheimer's Disease
- Fractures and Falls
- Talking with Your Doctor
- Nursing Homes: Making the Right Choice
- Choosing a Doctor
- Making Your Printed Health Materials Senior Friendly

National Patient Safety Agency
http://www.archive.npsa.nhs.uk/pleaseask/beinformed

Consumer fact sheets:

- Top 10 tips for safer patients
- Inpatients—About Staying in Hospital
- Medicines—Taking Them Safely
- Children—Easing Your Worries
- Relatives—Being Involved

National Patient Safety Foundation
http://www.npsf.org

- Ask Me 3™, three simple but essential questions that patients should ask their providers in every health care interaction

Sentara Healthcare Patient Safety Tips and Video
http://www.sentara.com/Sentara/PatientVisitorInfo/
PatientSafety/SafetyTips/

Virginians Improving Patient Care and Safety
http://www.vipcs.org/index.htm

Consumer fact sheets and brochures:

- Be Involved in Your Health Care: Tips to Help Prevent Medical Errors (Spanish version available)
- Tips on preventing medical errors related to medicines, hospital stays, surgery, home health, and other health services

Washington State Medical Association
http://www.wsma.org

Consumer brochures:

- Help Us Help You! Your Role in Safe Care
- 6 Ways to a Safer Hospital Stay
- The More We Know, the More We Can Help
- Handwashing Keeps Everyone Healthy

Yale-New Haven Hospital Tips for Staying Safe in the Hospital
http://www.ynhh.org/choice/safety.html

Government and Not-for-Profit Groups

American Hospital Association (AHA)
http://www.aha.org

This national organization represents and serves all types of hospitals, health care networks, and their patients and communities. To help hospitals become more patient and family focused in their care practices, the AHA partnered with the Institute for Family-Centered Care to produce "Strategies for Leadership: Patient- and Family Centered Care." The AHA also has produced a consumer fact sheet entitled "Patient Care Partnership: Understanding Expectations, Rights and Responsibilities" (available in multiple languages).

American Medical Association (AMA)
http://www.ama-assn.org/go/patientsafety

With its Making Strides in Safety® program, the AMA is helping physicians help patients by encouraging physician leadership and involvement in improving patient care.

American Society for Healthcare Risk Management, American Hospital Association

http://www.ashrm.org

A professional society for health care risk management professionals and those responsible for the process of making and carrying out decisions that will promote high-quality care, maintain a safe environment, and preserve human and financial resources in health care organizations. This organization published the white paper "Perspective on Disclosure of Unanticipated Outcome Information" (2001).

Institute for Healthcare Improvement

http://www.ihi.org

A not-for-profit organization created to help lead the improvement of health care systems to increase continuously their quality and value. The group sponsors initiatives intended to increase the role of patients and their families in health services.

National Patient Safety Agency

http://www.npsa.nhs.uk

This independent body coordinates the safety improvement efforts of all those involved in health care in the United Kingdom. Public involvement in safety improvement is a major initiative for the organization.

National Patient Safety Foundation

http://www.npsf.org

The National Patient Safety Foundation serves as a resource for individuals and organizations committed to improving the safety of patients. One of the goals of the organization is to raise public awareness about health care safety.

National Resource Centre for Consumer Participation in Health
http://www.participateinhealth.org.au

Australian organization that provides information on
consumer feedback and participation methodologies
and assists health care organizations in developing,
implementing, and evaluating consumer participation
methods and models.

Partnering for Patient Empowerment through Community
Awareness
http://www.galter.northwestern.edu/ppeca/index.htm

This collaboration among patient safety advocates, health
sciences librarians, health care institutions, and public
libraries developed a tool kit that can be used by libraries
to develop a patient safety partnership and awareness
program in their community.

Partnership for Patient Safety
http://www.p4ps.org

A patient-centered initiative focused on improving the
safety of health care through consumer involvement and a
systems approach.

Society for Healthcare Consumer Advocacy, American Hospital
Association
http://www.shca-aha.org

The Society for Healthcare Consumer Advocacy seeks to
advance health care consumer advocacy by supporting
the role of professionals who represent and advocate for
consumers across the health care continuum.

Whatcom County (WA) Pursuing Perfection Project
http://www.patientpowered.org

> The Whatcom County Pursuing Perfection Project began
> with the goal of perfecting care to patients by transforming
> the healthcare system. Its aims were to demonstrate that
> improved access to care, increased patient self-management
> and satisfaction, and decreased medication errors associated
> with care at different points in the health care system were
> all realistic and achievable goals. It is now an international
> effort with more than thirteen participating communities,
> including sites in Denmark, Sweden, and England as well as
> seven U.S. sites.

World Alliance for Patient Safety
http://www.who.int/patientsafety/en/

> The World Alliance for Patient Safety was formed by the
> World Health Organization to coordinate, disseminate,
> and accelerate improvements in patient safety worldwide.
> Its Patients for Patient Safety initiative emphasizes the
> central role patients and consumers can play in efforts to
> improve the quality and safety of health care around the
> world.

Patient- and Family-Centered Care Organizations

Institute for Family-Centered Care
http://www.familycenteredcare.org

> The mission of the Institute for Family-Centered Care is to
> advance the understanding and practice of family-centered
> care. The institute has developed several resources for
> health care professionals, including an assessment tool
> that can be used to evaluate the degree to which the cur-
> riculum, culture, and educational approach of a medical
> education program is likely to foster the competencies and
> attitudes necessary to practice family-centered care.

Planetree

http://www.planetree.org

The Planetree model of health care is patient centered rather than provider focused and is committed to improving medical care from the patient's perspective. It empowers patients and families through information and education and encourages "healing partnerships" with caregivers.

Consumer Groups

Consumers Advancing Patient Safety
http://www.patientsafety.org/

This consumer-led organization is a collective voice for individuals, families, and healers who wish to prevent harm in healthcare encounters through partnership and collaboration. The group partners with healthcare professionals, researchers, hospitals and other healthcare service organizations, government agencies, accreditors, educators, and others to promote the consumer perspective in patient safety.

Parents of Infants and Children with Kernicterus
http://www.PICKonline.org

This group was organized in late 2000 by a group of mothers of children with severe cerebral palsy resulting from kernicterus, a condition caused by excessive bilirubin levels in newborns. Parents of Infants and Children with Kernicterus has helped to create awareness about kernicterus and strategies for preventing this avoidable patient injury.

Patients Association
http://www.patients-association.com

A U.K. consumer group that publishes *Patient Voice* magazine (back issues available online) and offers advice to consumers on how to create better patient-practitioner partnerships.

P.U.L.S.E. (Persons United Limiting Substandards and Errors in Health Care)

http://www.pulseamerica.org

National consumer group geared toward education and support. The Web sites of state groups include some consumer-directed medical error prevention resources.

Products/Books

American Hospital Association

http://www.aha.org

- *Disclosure of Medical Errors: Demonstrated Strategy to Enhance Communication* (video) (2001), produced by the American Society for Healthcare Risk Management
- *Essentials of Patient Education* (2006), by Susan Bastable

B & R Publishing

http://www.patientjournal.com

Publisher of a patient journal designed for hospitalized patients and their families to record important medical information, physician names, medications, tests and procedures, and so on. The journal is intended to guide the patient through a hospital stay, beginning with admittance through the diagnostic and treatment regimen and finally discharge.

Joint Commission Resources

http://www.jcrinc.com

- *Patients as Partners: How to Involve Patients and Families in Their Own Care* (2006), by Meghan McGreevey

Jossey-Bass/John Wiley & Sons
http://www.josseybass.com

Books for health care professionals:

- *Advancing Health Literacy: A Framework for Understanding and Action* (2006), by Christina Zarcadoolas, Andrew Pleasant, and David S. Greer
- *Cultural Competence in Health Care* (2002), edited by Anne Rundle, Maria Carvalho, and Mary Robinson
- *Through the Patient's Eyes: Understanding and Promoting Patient-Centered Care* (2002), edited by Margaret Gerteis, Susan Edgman-Levitan, Jennifer Daley, and Thomas L. Delbanco
- *Putting Patients First: Designing and Practicing Patient-Centered Care* (2003), edited by Susan Frampton, Laura Gilpin, and Patrick Charmel
- *What Do I Say? Communicating Intended or Unanticipated Outcomes in Obstetrics* (2003), by James R. Woods and Fay A. Rozovsky

Savard System
http://www.drsavard.com

The Savard System empowers patients to be their own best health advocates and provides tools for patients to become informed and involved. The system grew out of Dr. Marie Savard's three decades of experience as a medical practitioner, first as a nurse and then as a general internist and primary care physician.

- *How to Save Your Own Life* (Warner Books, 2000), by Marie Savard
- *The Savard Health Record: A Six-Step System for Managing Your Healthcare* (Time-Life Books, 2000), by Marie Savard

Miscellaneous books for health care consumers available from various book retailers, including Amazon.com:

- *American Medical Association Guide to Talking to Your Doctor* (John Wiley & Sons, 2001), by the American Medical Association
- *Confessions of a Professional Hospital Patient: A Humorous First-Person Account of How to Survive a Hospital Stay and Escape with Your Life, Dignity and a Sense of Humor* (1st Books Library, 2001), by Michael Weiss
- *How to Get Out of the Hospital Alive: A Guide to Patient Power* (John Wiley & Sons, 1998), by Sheldon Blau and Elaine Shimberg
- *How to Survive Your Hospital Stay* (Center Press, 1998), by Judy Burger Crane
- *Internal Bleeding: The Truth Behind America's Terrifying Epidemic of Medical Mistakes* (RuggedLand Books, 2004), by Robert Wachter and Kaveh Shojania.
- *Making Informed Medical Decisions: Where to Look and How to Use What You Find* (O'Reilly & Associates, 2000), by Lucy Thomas, Nancy Oster, and Darol Joseff
- *So You're Having a Heart Cath and Angioplasty* (John Wiley & Sons, 2003), by Magnus Ohman, Gail Cox, Stephen Fort, and Victoria K. Folger
- *The Intelligent Patient's Guide to the Doctor-Patient Relationship: Learning How to Talk So Your Doctor Will Listen* (Oxford University Press, 1998), by Barbara Korsch and Caroline Harding
- *YOU: The Smart Patient: An Insider's Handbook for Getting the Best Treatment* (Free Press, 2006), by Michael Roizen and Mehmet Oz

Index